Life Sciences Monographs   *1*

Life Sciences Monographs

Editor: G. Raspé

Associate Editor: S. Bernhard

Technical Assistance:

H. Schmidt

Life Sciences Monographs 1

International Symposium
on the Treatment
of Carcinoma of the Prostate
Berlin, November 13 to 15, 1969

Editors: G. Raspé and W. Brosig
Associate Editors: S. Bernhard and H. Baumgärtel

Moderator:
W. E. Goodwin

This volume is sponsored by
Schering AG, D-1 Berlin 65, Müllerstraße 170—172

Pergamon Press · Vieweg

Oxford · Edinburgh · New York
Toronto · Sidney · Braunschweig

Pergamon Press Ltd., Headington Hill Hall, Oxford
Pergamon Press (Scotland) Ltd., 2 & 3 Teviot Place, Edinburgh 1
Pergamon Press Inc., Maxwell House, Fairview Park, Elmsford, New York 10523
Pergamon of Canada Ltd., 207 Queen's Quay West, Toronto 1
Pergamon Press (Aust.) Pty. Ltd., 19a Boundary Street, Rushcutters Bay,
N. S. W. 2011, Australia
Vieweg + Sohn GmbH, Burgplatz 1, Braunschweig

Editorial Assistance: *Bernhard Lewerich*

ISBN 0 08 017572 4   (Pergamon)

ISBN 3 528 07811 1   (Vieweg)

1971

Set by Friedr. Vieweg + Sohn GmbH, Braunschweig
Printed by E. Hunold, Braunschweig
Bookbinder: W. Langelüddecke, Braunschweig
Cover design: Herbert W. Kapitzki, Frankfurt
Printed in Germany-West

Table of Contents

Introductions

W. Brosig and W. E. Goodwin*)

Urologische Klinik und Poliklinik im Klinikum Steglitz der Freien Universität Berlin, Germany

*) Division of Urology, The Center of Health Sciences, University of California,
Los Angeles, USA

W. Brosig: Ladies and Gentlemen! Dear colleagues from abroad and Germany! It is a pleasure and a great honour to welcome so many distinguished guests and experts from the whole world. This was made possible by the generosity of the Schering AG here in Berlin, which has unselfishly created the conditions which have enabled us to undertake this conference. I repeat unselfishly because the final results of this symposium may not ultimately prove to be in the economic interests of the company. Further support was given by Asta AG, Brackwede.

The real reason for arranging this meeting was the uncertainty and confusion in the treatment of carcinoma of the prostate which was caused by a paper published in the Journal of Urology in October 1967. In this paper 14 American hospitals and clinics pooled their statistics on over 2000 patients with carcinoma. The 5 year survival rate of patients treated with orchiectomy and placebo, was compared. Now I will read you the summary of this paper: "In this series the average patient with prostatic carcinoma did not derive much clinical benefit from immediate treatment with either orchiectomy or a 5 mg daily oral dose of stilboestrol, unless the cancer was causing serious problems. The excess mortality associated with oestrogen therapy, the psychological trauma of orchiectomy, the adverse affects of the placebo itself and the clinical benefits obtained when patients with progressing disease were shifted from placebo to more active treatments, all combine to suggest that therapy with oestrogen or orchiectomy should be withheld until the patient's symptoms are so severe as to requne relief. Treatment earlier in the disease is not likely to help and may cause considerable damage. Either oestrogen alone or orchiectomy alone provided all the clinical benefits of the 2 in combination. The bad results are due to cardiovascular diseases, caused by the oestrogen treatment. 50 % of the diseased did not succumb due to the carcinoma but due to the cardiovascular or other diseases."

In general the high percentage of the 5-year survival rates in the published paper is surprising, especially if you look at the old statistics of *Baum* and *Nesbit* and other papers, including our own experiences with hormone therapy and castration. The rate in our cases is, for example, 40 % if there are no metastases and 20 % in patients with metastases. This number corresponds to the results of *Baum* and *Nesbit*.

The aim of this symposium should be to resolve the doubts and uncertainty in the treatment of carcinoma of the prostate and formulate a new policy for treatment in the future. For this purpose we have invited the most important experts in this field. Some of them will read a short paper on selected subjects. These papers should provide the basis for profound discussions. I would like to ask those who are not named in the first program, but who are not less important than the others, to take full part in these discussions.

I give the chair to *Willard E. Goodwin,* who will work as a moderator.

W. E. Goodwin: We will now have the introductory papers. The first paper this morning will be given by Dr. *Hodges* on *"The basis of hormonal treatment"*. I am going then to ask Dr. *Salloch*, Dr. *Williams* and Dr. *Brock* to give us their talks about the pharmacological aspects of the treatment of cancer of the prostate.

Then we will hear from Dr. *Mostofi* on the pathology of carcinoma of the prostate.

Basis of Hormonal Treatment of Prostatic Cancer

C. V. Hodges

Division of Urology, University of Oregon Medical School Portland, Oregon, USA

Summary: Reports of benefit accruing to patients with prostatic obstruction who underwent orchiectomy were published in 1895, and 1896. Indubitably, some of these were examples of prostatic carcinoma. Further progress awaited the demonstration by *Huggins* and his group that the prostate gland in dogs was stimulated by androgens and inhibited by orchiectomy or administration of estrogens. The application of these principles to patients with prostatic cancer led to similar findings and constituted the basis for the current hormonal treatment regimens.

Prostatic carcinoma was not recognized definitely before the early 19th century. Prior to that time, it was confused with other forms of prostatic enlargement. *Langstaff* [1] in 1817, was probably the first individual to report an authentic case of prostatic cancer. *Thompson* [2] discussed cancer of the prostate in 1858, reporting 23 cases; this was the first large study of cancer of the prostate in the literature. Reports of attempts to cure prostatic cancer by surgical means include several famous names: *Billroth, Wyss, Kocher, Harrison, Kuster, Von Recklinghausen, Courvoisier* and *Young*. It was recognized early that the percentage of patients who were suitable for surgical treatment of prostatic cancer was extremely small.

The hypothesis advanced by *White* [3] in 1895 was that enlargement of the prostate bears the same relationship to the testes as fibroid disease of the uterus does to the ovaries. He reported a series of 111 patients operated on for symptoms of marked prostatic obstruction with marked elevation of residual urine. Bilateral orchiectomy was carried out on all patients with an overall improvement of 75 %. There were 20 deaths for a mortality rate of 18 %; however, many of these patients were extremely ill from uremia and were operated on in desperation. No biopsies were made; the diagnosis was made by rectal examination. Four of 111 patients were described as having an extremely hard prostate gland; these patients all improved dramatically.

Cabot [4] in 1896 reviewed the evidence for the effect of castration on the enlarged prostate. "Castration would seem to be especially efficacious in cases of large tense prostates when the obstruction is due to pressure of the lateral lobes upon the urethra. Castration is of but little use in myomatous and fibrous prostates."

Manuscript received: 13 November 1969

Beatson [5] discovered in 1896 that bilateral oophorectomy had a beneficial effect on cancer of the breast in women. He stated "we must look in the female to the ovaries as the seat of the exciting cause of carcinoma, certainly of the mamma, in all probability of the female generative organs generally and possibly of the rest of the body."

The scientific basis for the hormonal control of cancer of the prostate may be said to have been initiated in 1932 when *Lacassagne* [6] demonstrated that injections of estrone caused the development of mammary cancer in males of a special strain of mice. It remained for *Huggins* et al. [7] to demonstrate the dependancy of benign and malignant enlargements of the prostate gland on the androgens of the testis. The dog was chosen as the experimental animal since it developed spontaneous prostatic hypertrophy, which is similar to that in man. It was necessary to devise a preparation which would allow the longterm study of the effects of various agents on the prostate gland. The preparation was based on *Eckhart's* [8] method of ligation of the bladder neck to prevent the passage of urine into the urethra, and a cannula in the urethra to deliver the prostatic secretion, as modified by *Farrell* [9], who divided the prostatovesical junction, in-folded both ends and created an anastomosis between the fundus of the bladder and the prepuce; a week later, a fistula of the urethra was formed in the perineum. Modification used by *Huggins* employed the separation of bladder and prostate with insertion of a brass cannula into the bladder for permanent diversion of the urine. The isolated prostate then drained into the urethra and, after division of the prepuce, a collecting flask could be suspended around the shaft of the penis for collections of prostatic fluid. Pilocarpine, 6 mg., in saline, was given intravenously as the standard stimulating cholinergic drug. Collections were for hourly periods following pilocarpine administration.

The findings essential to our discussion today are in the summary: "The rate of prostatic atrophy following castration was determined, and cessation of secretion occurred in 7–23 days. The restoration of prostatic fluid in castrate dogs following daily injections of testosterone propionate followed a smooth curve to form a plateau which was interrupted occasionally by prolonged elevations with returns to the established level. The prostate having been reconstructed, the dosage of androgenic material injected could be greatly reduced without causing a decrease in secretion. Ablation of the thyroid and parathyroid glands had no significant influence on prostatic secretion. Hyperthyroidism caused a secretory depression interrupted with returns to normal levels". It was also noted that in a castrated dog whose prostate was maintained by daily injections of testosterone propionate, removal of one adrenal showed no effect on prostatic fluid output. But a slight depression of prostatic output followed removal of the second adrenal gland.

Subsequent studies by *Huggins* and *Clark* [10] resulted in several interesting findings. Cystic hyperplasia was found in the prostate glands of aging dogs, associated with worn teeth, lens opacities, and testicular tumors. These cystic glands in the older dogs produced less prostatic fluid after stimulation than did those of young, vigorous dogs. Orchiectomy caused a marked decrease in prostatic secretions, reaching the lowest level 7—23 days after operation. In the normal prostate, the tall columnar epithelium of the prostatic alveoli and ducts decreased in size, and within two months consisted of closely grouped low basophilic cells, stratified in places. There was no appreciable secretion from the gland unless the epithelium was of columnar type. At three months, all of the epithelium was flat. Small lamina were seen in most of the acini, but some of the spaces had completely disappeared. In cystic hyperplasia, castration showed a very similar effect which continued for at least three months. Administration of testosterone propionate resulted in a reversal of atrophy, both grossly and microscopically.

Injected estrogens caused slight increase in the weight of the prostate gland of puppies. Squamous epithelial metaplasia of the urethra was noted. Estrogens after orchiectomy again resulted in stratified squamous epithelium. The prostate glands of two senile dogs injected with one milligram of stilbestrol daily, increased in size. The acini were lined with flattened epithelium and distended with leukocytes. There was intense squamous metaplasia. In old dogs, whose prostate glands were actively secreting, stilbestrol injections caused a significant decrease in secretory volume. In dogs with prostatic hyperplasia receiving stilbestrol injections, the prostate gland was shrunken in size, due to reduction in size of prostatic epithelium and of the prostatic cysts and acini. When a castrate dog, whose prostatic secretion had been steadily increasing due to daily injections of testosterone propionate, 10 mg., received increasing daily doses of stilbestrol, it was found that this characteristic rising curve became a plateau and that an increased dosage of estrogen caused decrease in the amount of secretion. Prostate glands of those dogs receiving both testosterone and stilbestrol did not atrophy. There were combined effects of both the androgen and the estrogen on cell appearance.

An objective method of determining the activity of prostatic cancer was found in the use of acid and alkaline serum phosphatase. *Kutscher* and *Wolbergs* [11] discovered that acid phosphatase is found in the prostate of adult human males in amounts greatly in excess of those in other organs. *Gutman* and *Gutman* [12] described the elevation of serum acid phosphatase in patients with metastatic prostatic cancer. *Kay* [13] showed that increased alkaline phosphatase levels in serum may be due to increased osteoblastic activity. *Huggins* and *Hodges* [14] found that the *King* and *Armstrong* method for determining serum phosphatases was adaptable to the estimation of large numbers of serum specimens. This method was used to follow the progress of patients who underwent castration, estrogen and androgen administration after the diagnosis of metastatic prostatic cancer had been made, as well as a group of normal men and men with prostatic hypertrophy. Normal values were established at 3.25 plus or minus 1.37 KA units/100 cc. serum for acid phosphatase, and 7.9 plus or minus 2.1 units/100 cc. for alkaline phosphatase. In a group of 25 men with roentgenologic evidence of metastatic carcinoma to the bony pelvis, both alkaline and acid phosphatases were increased above normal in 19 cases. Only alkaline phosphatase was increased in two cases and both values were within normal limits in four cases. In prostatic cancer with marked elevation of acid phosphatase, castration or injection of large amounts of estrogen caused a sharp reduction of this enzyme toward the normal range. Alkaline phosphatase values rose following castration and then decreased, but more slowly than acid phosphatase. In three patients with prostatic cancer, androgen injection caused a sharp rise in serum acid phosphatase. In one case following cessation of androgen there was a decrease of the acid phosphatase followed by a secondary spontaneous rise. The conclusion was "prostatic cancer is influenced by androgenic activity in the body. At least with respect to serum phosphatases, disseminated carcinoma of the prostate is inhibited by eliminating androgens, through castration, or neutralization of the activity by estrogen injection. Cancer of the prostate is activated by androgen injections [11]". In a subsequent paper, *Huggins, Stevens,* and *Hodges* [15] reported that 21 consecutive patients had been treated by castration for far-advanced or metastatic carcinoma of the prostate. "Four patients died at eight months after the operation; in two cases, the operation was done too recently to allow deductions as to its efficacy, and in fifteen cases, appreciable clinical improvement occurred. The objective evidence of benefit after orchiectomy consisted of a great decrease in the levels of serum phosphatase in all but two cases, an increase in weight (and appetite), an increase in the red cells of the peripheral blood, and decrease in the amount of pain, shrinkage of the primary lesion, increased density of the metastatic lesion, in the roentgenograms; and in one case, improvement in neurologic signs of compression of the cauda equina by metastases. The improvement was greater than we have observed in any case in which far-advanced or metastatic cancer was treated any other way. It is certain that in many cases, regression of the neoplasm is not complete."

References

[1] *Langstaff, G.:* Cases of fungus haematodes. Medico-Chirurgical, Trans., London. Longman, Hurst, Rees, Orme, and Brown. 1817. vol. 8, part I, pp. 279–288. (This later became the Royal Med. Chir. Soc. Trans.)

[2] *Thompson, H.:* The enlarged prostate, its pathology and treatment. London, John Churchill, 1858. pp. 212–229.

[3] *White, J. W.:* The results of double castration in hypertrophy of the prostate. Annals of Surgery **22**, 1, 1895.

[4] *Cabot, A. T.:* The question of castration for enlarged prostate. Annals of Surgery **24**, 265, 1896.

[5] *Beatson, G. T.:* On the treatment of inoperable cases of carcinoma of the mamma: Suggestions for a new method of treatment with illustrative cases. Lancet **2**, 104, 1896.

[6] *Lacassagne, A.:* Compt. Rend. **195**, 630, 1932.

[7] *Huggins, C., Masina, M. H., Eichelberger, L.* and *Wharton, J. D.:* Quantitative Studies of Prostatic Secretion. I. Characteristics of the normal secretion; the influence of thyroid, suprarenal, and testis extirpation and androgen substitution on the prostatic output. J. Exp. Med. **70**, 543, 1939.

[8] *Eckhard, C.:* Beitr. Anat. U. Physiol. **3**, 155, 1863.

[9] *Farrell, J. I.:* Tr. Am. Ass'n. Genitourinary Surgeons **24**, 221, 1931.

[10] *Huggins, C.* and *Clark, P. J.:* Quantitative studies of prostatic secretion. II. The effect of castration and of estrogen injection of the normal and of the hyperplastic prostate glands of dogs. J. Exp. Med. **72**, 747, 1940.

[11] *Kutscher* and *Wolbergs:* Zeitschrift für Physiol. Chem. **236**, 237, 1935.

[12] *Gutman, A. B.* and *Gutman, E. B.:* An "Acid" phosphatase occurring in the serum of patients with metastasizing carcinoma of the prostate gland. J. Clin. Invest. **17**, 473, 1938.

[13] *Kay, H. D.:* Plasma phosphate in osteitis deformans and in other diseases of bone. J. Exp. Path. **10**, 253, 1929.

[14] *Huggins, C.* and *Hodges, C. V.:* Studies on Prostatic Cancer. I. The effect of castration, of estrogens and of androgens injection on serum phosphatase in metastatic carcinoma of the prostate. Cancer Res. **1**, 293, 1941.

[15] *Huggins, C., Stevens, R.* and *Hodges, C. V.:* Studies on Prostatic Cancer. II. The effects of castration on advanced carcinoma of the prostate gland. Arch. Surg. **43**, 209, 1941.

Hormonal Treatment of Cancer of the Prostate Pharmacological Aspects

R. R. Salloch, F. Neumann and M. Kramer

Schering AG, Berlin, Germany

Summary : At the prostate of castrated Sprague-Dawley rats,estrogens do not influence the androgen action, i.e.,increase of ventral prostate weight. In castrated plus hypophysectomized rats,a distinct estrogen-androgen antagonism at the prostate can be demonstrated.

Estrogen treatment increases the prolactin (LTH) secretion via a positive feed-back mechanism. It is known that exogenous prolactin maintains and potentiates the growth of the prostate in castrated and hypophysectomized rats in synergism with androgens. Prolactin substitution seems to overcome the estrogen-androgen antagonism in castrated plus hypophysectomized rats. We advance the tentative hypothesis that in castrated rats under estrogen and androgen influence most likeley two different estrogen actions occur simultaneously : centrally increased LTH-secretion and the antagonistic action at the prostate level. It seems that one effect exceeds the other one.

The influence of the antiandrogen cypoterone acetate on the regulatory mechanisms of the hypophyseal-diencephalic system is shown, as well as its possible local efficiency at the prostate (see legend Fig. 13).

At this time, estrogens are still the therapy of choice in the treatment of cancer of the prostate. When a clinician speaks of "anti-androgen" therapy in carcinoma of the prostate, he usually refers to castration with subsequent estrogen medication. This brings the discussion to the following pharmacological aspects:

(1) What are the long-term effects of estrogen treatment on the pituitary diencephalic system?

(2) Is the prostate gland of rats a target organ for estrogens even though

(3) estrogens are definitely not antiandrogenic substances?

(4) What is the mechanism by which anti-androgens interfere with hormonal regulations?

The following illustrations are taken from studies by *Huggins and Clark* [20], *Goodwin*, *Scott* and others [15], who demonstrated in dogs a dose-related estrogen androgen antagonism (The parameter was the prostatic secretion) [15, 20, 21, 27, 46]. Figure 1 shows the experiment with a castrated dog.

Manuscript received : 19 January 1970

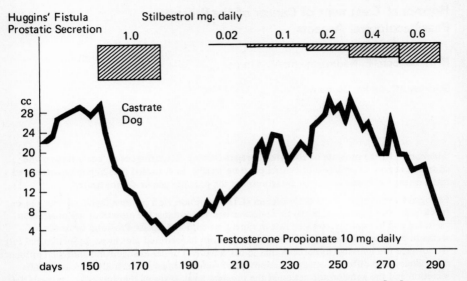

Fig. 1. Estrogen-androgen antagonism in the castrated dog (prostatic secretion) [20].

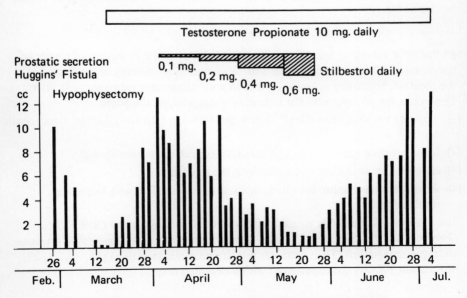

Fig. 2. Estrogen-androgen antagonism in the hypophysectomized dog (prostatic secretion) [15].

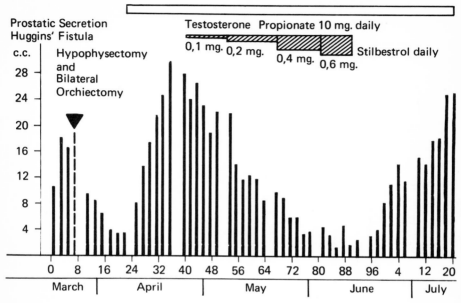

Fig. 3. Estrogen-androgen antagonism in the hypophysectomized-castrated dog (prostatic secretion) [46].

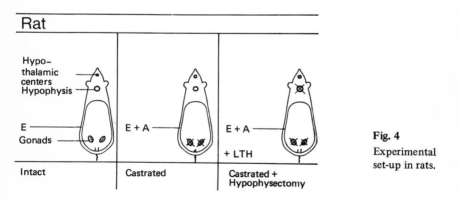

Fig. 4
Experimental set-up in rats.

This antagonism is manifest in hypophysectomized dogs (Fig. 2) as well as in hypophysectomized and castrated animals (Fig. 3).

Most of the studies in this field have been performed on rats, and the following experiments were also carried out on Sprague-Dawley rats.

The animals shown in Fig. 4 were treated with androgens in combination with estrogens and LTH (prolactin).

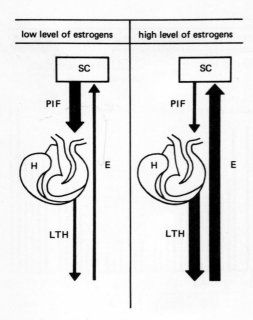

Fig. 5
Positive feed-back mechanism of
LTH (prolactin) and estrogens.

By a central inhibitory mechanism, estrogens are known to reduce LH (ICSH) output in intact animals, thereby lowering the androgen levels, and comparable activity has been demonstrated in humans [1, 13, 42, 44, 45].

Nevertheless, under prolonged estrogen medication, the anti-LH activity declines gradually, even if the estrogen dose is maintained [17, 18, 28]. *Hohlweg* interpretes this process as a desensitization in the pituitary-diencephalic system, whereby the sensitivity of hypothalamic centers to estrogen is lowered to the point where LH secretion can no longer be inhibited or the estrogen dosage has to be increased more and more.

Another consequence of prolonged estrogen medication in rats and other rodents (rabbits, mice, guinea pigs) is a reversible hyperplasia of the adenohypophysis, which constitutes the morphologic substrate of overstimulated prolactin secretion. An increase of weight under estrogen medication in short-time experiments is well known, too. In contrast to other gonadotropins, a positive feed-back mechanism exists between estrogens and prolactin output and secretion [2, 23, 29, 30, 31, 35].

There is substantial evidence that prolactin synthesis and release in mammals are chronically depressed by a hypothalamic prolactin-inhibiting factor. The LTH-secretion of the pituitary increases under estrogens, presumably by inhibition of the synthesis of the PIF [29, 30].

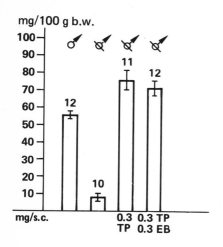

Fig. 6

No estrogen-androgen antagonism in castrated rats (ventral prostate weight).

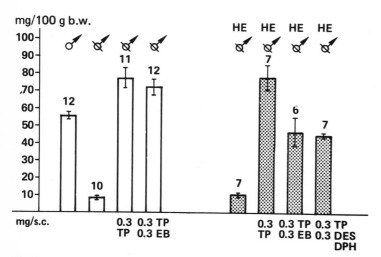

Fig. 7. Estrogen-androgen antagonism in hypophysectomized-castrated rats (ventral prostate weight).

Probably, gynecomastia in males is in part an effect of elevated prolactin levels under prolonged estrogen treatment, also occurring in patients receiving long-term therapy with drugs acting on the diencephalon and inhibiting the prolactin inhibiting factor, such as chlorpromazine (Atosil) and chlordiazepoxide (Librium) [2].

Estrogens, whether stilbestrol or estradiol, are incapable of suppressing exogenous testosterone in the prostate of castrated rats [10, 24].

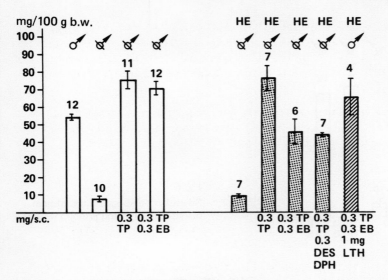

Fig. 8. Inhibition of estrogen-androgen antagonism in hypophysectomized-castrated rat by LTH (ventral prostate weight).

Figure 6 illustrates our studies on castrated rats. Juvenile castrated rats were given a 7-day estrogen and androgen combination treatment following a 7-day involutional period. The parameter is the ventral prostate. Even under excessive estrogen doses, there are hardly any differences in the results, compared to testosterone propionat-substituted controls.

Figure 7 shows a distinctive contrast to these results.

The experimental design and the dosages are identical, except that the animals are also hypophysectomized. There is a clear-cut estrogen-androgen antagonism here; the estrogens used in the experiment, estradiol benzoate and diethylstilbestrol diphosphate, act in the same manner.

The LTH-secretion of the pituitary, as already mentioned, increases under estrogens.

Therefore, it was indicated to examine the role of LTH in our experimental model and it was found that LTH-replacement seems to inhibit the effect of estrogens in hypophysectomized and castrated animals at the prostate level. In spite of the small number of animals the statistical analysis was possible (V-test).

It is known that prolactin, most probably in synergism with androgens, maintains and potentiates the growth of the prostate in castrated and hypophysectomized rats [2, 6, 7, 16].

In rats which were not hypophysectomized, estrogens gave a result which was paradoxical at first sight. However, if one takes into consideration that two different estrogen actions took place simultaneously — centrally increased LTH secretion and the antagonistic action at the prostate level — it is understandable that one effect may mask the other one.

In this context, it may be referred to *Scott* and others who noticed earlier that the effects of estrogens on the (androgen-dependent segments of) the prostate varied from species to species [3, 20, 24, 43, 46, 47, 54].

It has been shown that an anti-androgen like cyproterone abolishes almost all effects of androgens on accessory sexual organs, thus acting in analogy to castration in a dose dependent way. In addition it was shown in parabiotically joined rats that the secretion of LH and FSH is increased by way of occupation of androgen-sensitive receptors within the central nervous system.

This was supported by results published by *Bloch* and *Davidson* [8] who showed corroborating effects by implantation techniques with very small amounts of cyproterone within the hypothalamus [5, 8, 37–41].

Cyproterone acetate does not give the same effect because it has not only anti-androgenic but also a distinctive progestational property.

So far, more than 200 antiandrogenic substances, both steroids and non-steroids, have been discovered. Fig. 9 shows two of these antiandrogens, derivatives of hydroxyprogesterone.

(On the left there is cyproterone, and right, its acetate, esterified in position C_{17}, the most potent anti-androgen known so far.)

We share the view of other authors [33, 34, 52, 53] that *in vivo* these anti-androgens act at the level of the receptors by way of a competitive antagonism to testosterone; still, *in vitro* studies point to other sites of action [4, 12]. We would rather not attempt an interpretation of these *in vitro* findings, since none of us is a biochemist, and it would be presumptuous to venture into this area.

Figure 10 and 11 illustrate the castration-like effect of cyproterone acetate.

Anti-androgens antagonize the effect not only of testicular androgens, but also of dehydroepiandrosterone and androstenedione [51]. *Tullner* [49] and other authors [9, 32] have shown that the (ventral) prostate of castrated rats may be maintained and stimulated by ACTH treatment. The weight of the adrenal glands in male rats tends to increase after castration, an effect which is potentiated by estrogens [10, 14, 22, 48].

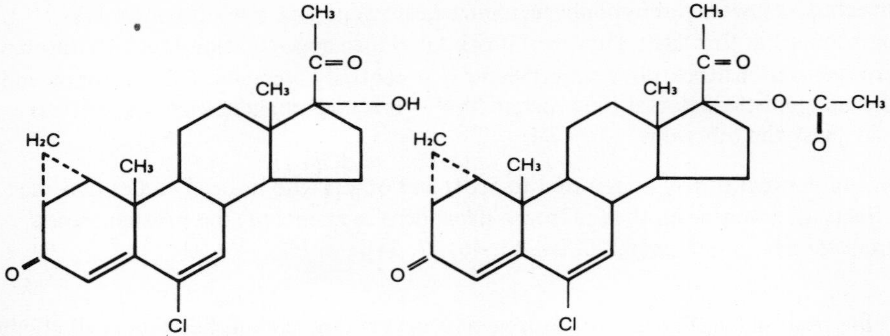

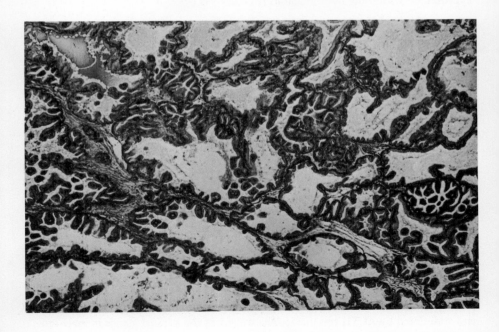

Fig. 9. Cyproterone and Cyroterone acetate.
Left: 1,2α-Methylene-6-chloro-$\Delta^{4,6}$-pregnadiene-17α-ol-3,20-dione (= Cyproterone).
Right: 1,2α-Methylene-6-chloro-$\Delta^{4,6}$-pregnadiene-17α-ol-3,20-dione-17α-acetate
(= Cyproterone acetate).

Fig. 10. Normal dog prostate.

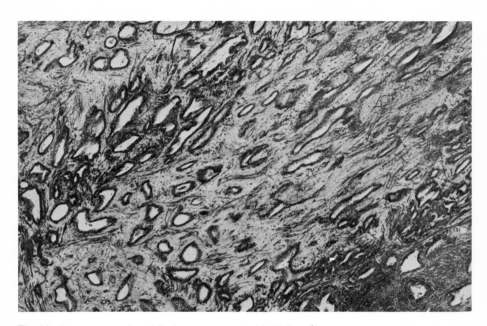

Fig. 11. Dog prostate after daily i. m. treatment with 10.0 mg/kg cyproterone acetate for 30 days.

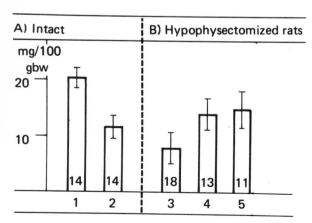

CYPAC 3 mg/100 g bw/d, s.c. and ACTH
(800 m U) 100 g bw/d/s.c
Duration of treatment 14 days

Fig. 12

Adrenal weight of male rats and cyproterone acetate. 1 Intact control, 2 Cyproterone acetate, 3 Hypophysectomized control, 4 Hypophysectomy + ACTH, 5 Hypophysectomy + ACTH + Cyproterone acetate.

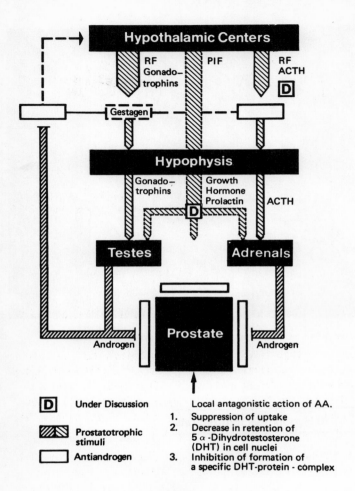

Fig. 13. The action of cyproterone acetate at hypothalamus and prostate of rats.

Left: Anti-androgens without partial effects result in a blockade of the androgen-sensitive receptors in the diencephalon in male animals, causing an increase in gonadotropin production and secretion. Cyproterone acetate, with its progestational side effects, simultaneously inhibits the gonadotropic function of the hypophyseal − diencephalic system.

Right: Cyproterone acetate causes a definite inhibition of the corticotropic function in the hypophyseal − diencephalic system with a decrease in ACTH-secretion.

Middle: It is not yet clear whether cyproterone acetate influences the release of prolactin (LTH) or growth hormone.

Bottom: Anti-androgens competitively inhibit the effects of androgens on the receptors (prostate, testis, diencephalon). The effect of cyproterone acetate on the molecular level postulated by *Fang* and *Liao* [12] is indicated at the bottom right.

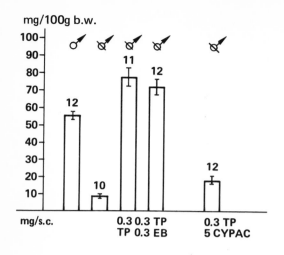

Fig. 14

See Fig. 6 anti-androgenic action not of estrogen, but of cyproterone acetate.

Doménico and *Neumann* [11] investigated the effect of cyproterone acetate on the weight of the adrenal glands in male rats (Fig. 12).

The adrenal weight loss under cyproterone acetate in hypophysectomized rats could be reserved by the concomitant administration of exogenous ACTH (800 m.U. alone, shown in column 4, and with cyproterone acetate added, in column 5). From this, we derived the conclusion that the effect of antiandrogens on the adrenal function does not represent a direct effect on the organ itself, but rather an inhibition of the corticotropic function in the pituitary-diencephalic system.

Neri [34] supported our findings with the adrenal glands. However, it might be that this ACTH depressing action is species-specific and not necessarily it might apply for the human. It should be mentioned in support of this hypothesis that different gestagens (e.g., 6-methyl-17-acetoxy-progesterone) behaved similar to the cyproterone acetate in rats, but different in the human where these effects were not observed [19, 33, 34]. Clinical trials with cyproterone acetate coming up now are in line with these suggestions [25].

The scheme in Figure 13 illustrates our interpretations of the action of cyproterone acetate at the prostate level of rats.

We might stress purposely another time that the action of cyproterone acetate shows a fundamental difference as compared to estrogen in rats (Fig. 14).

Within our experimental design the (estrogen-induced) LH (ICSH) inhibition makes sense only if the target organ, the interstitial cells of the testis are present.

Estrogens stimulate the LTH secretion rather extensively, and, simultaneously there is an increase of the ACTH secretion too [10, 14, 22, 48]. These enhanced hypophyseal secretions could turn out into an additional stimulus within the prostate gland, an effect which is definitely undesirable from the therapeutical view-point.

In contrast, anti-androgens are specific in their action and it seems unlikely that they favor LTH or ACTH secretions.

Furthermore, anti-androgens inhibit androgens by competitive antagonism at the target organ's level, in this case the prostate gland, regardless from which structure they originate.

As of now, there is no generally accepted definition of the term 'antihormone' but in our opinion estrogens have positively no anti-androgenic power whatsoever. We are obliged to explain our prostate data under estrogen influence in a different way. It might be wise to take into consideration that other mechanisms — e. g., antimitotic — might have been involved. It is therefore necessary to carry out further experiments to correlate these results.

References

[1] *Adler, A., H. Burger, J. Davis, A. Dulmanis, B. Hudson, G. Sarfaty* and *W. Straffon*: Brit. med. J. 1, 28 (1968).

[2] *Apostolakis, M.*: Vitamines and Hormones 26, 197 (1968).

[3] *Balogh, F.* and *Z. Szendröi*: "Cancer of the Prostate"Akademiai Kiado, Budapest 1968.

[4] *Belham, J. E., G. E. Neal*, and *D. C. Williams*: submitted for publication (1969).

[5] *von Berswordt-Wallrabe, R.*, and *F. Neumann*: Neuroendocrinology 3, 332 (1968).

[6] *von Berswordt-Wallrabe, R., U. Bielitz, W. Elger*, and *H. Steinbeck*: J. Urol. submitted for publication (1969).

[7] *von Berswordt-Wallrabe, R., H. Steinbeck, J. D. Hahn* and *W. Elger*: Experentia (Basel) 25, 533 (1969).

[8] *Bloch, G. J.* and *J. M. Davidson*: Science **155**, 593 (1967).

[9] *Davidson, C. S.* and *H. D. Moon*: Proc. Soc. exp. Biol. (N. Y.) **35**, 281 (1936).

[10] *Dörner, G.*: Wiss. Z. Humboldt-Universität Berlin Math. Nat. R. **XI**, 915 (1962).

[11] *Doménico, A.* and *F. Neumann*: 12. Symp. Dtsch. Ges. f. Endokrinologie, Wiesbaden, S. 312 (1966). Springer-Verlag, Berlin-Heidelberg-New York.

[12] *Fang, S.* and *S. Liao*: Molec. Pharmacol. in press (1970).

[13] *Forchielli, E., G. S. Rao, J. R. Sarda, N. B. Gibree, P. E. Pochi, J. S. Strauss* and *R. I. Dorfman*: Acta endocr. (Kbh). **50**, 51 (1965).

[14] *Gemzell, C. A.*: Acta endocr. (Kbh.) Suppl. **1**, 1 (1948).

[15] *Goodwin, D. A., D. S. Rasmussen-Taxdal, A. A. Ferreira* and *W. W. Scott*: J. Urol. **86/1**, 134 (1961).

[16] *Grayhack, J. T.*: Nat. Cancer Inst. Monograph **12**, 189 (1963).

[17] *Hohlweg, W.*: In: *Seitz-Amreich* (ed.): Biologie und Pathologie des Weibes. Urban und Schwarzenberg (1953).

[18] *Hohlweg, W.*: Dtsch. Gesundh.-Wes. **11**, 245 (1956).

[19] *Holub, D. A., F. H. Katz* and *J. W. Jailer*: Endocrinology **68**, 173 (1961).

[20] *Huggins, Ch.* and *P. J. Clark*: J. exp. Med. **72**, 747 (1940).

[21] *Huggins, Ch.* and *J. L. Sommer*: J. exp. Med. **97**, 663 (1953).

[22] *Jones, I. Ch.*: "The Adrenal Cortex", Univ. Press, Cambridge, p. 102 (1957).

[23] *Kanemutsu, S.* and *C. H. Sawyer*: Endocrinology **72**, 243 (1963).

[24] *Korenchewski, V.* and *M. Dennison*: J. Path. Bact. **41**, 323 (1935).

[25] *Laschet, U.*: pers. comm. (1969).

[26] *Lindner, A., I. Satke* and *O. Voelkel*: Wien. klin. Wschr. **65**, 789 (1953).

[27] *Marden, H. E.* jr., *J. T. Grayhack* and *W. W. Scott*: J. Urol. **73/4**, 703 (1955).

[28] *McCann, S. M.* and *Y. D. Ramirez*: Recent Progr. Hormone Res. **20**, 131 (1964).

[29] *Meites, J.*: In: *Martini, L.* and *W. F. Ganong* (ed.): Neuroendocrinology I, Acad. Press New York/London p. 669 (1966).

[30] *Meites, J.* and *Ch. S. Nicoll*: Amer. Rev. Physiol. **28**, 57 (1966).

[31] *Meites, J., Ch. S. Nicoll* and *P. K. Talwalker*: In: *Nalbandow, A. V.* (ed.): "Advances in Neuroendocrinology" Urbana (1963).

[32] *Nelson, W. O.*: Anat. Rec. Suppl. **81**, 97 (1941).

[33] *Neri, R. O., C. Casmer, W. V. Zeman, F. Fiedler* and *I. A. Tabachnik*: Endocrinology **82**, 311 (1968).

[34] *Neri, R. O., M. D. Monahan, J. G. Meyer, B. A. Afonso* and *I. A. Tabachnik*: Europ. J. Pharmacol. **1**, 438 (1967).

[35] *Neumann, F.*: unpublished (1968).

[36] *Neumann, F.* and *R. von Berswordt-Wallrabe*: J. Endocr. **35**, 363 (1966).

[37] *Neumann, F., R. von Berswordt-Wallrabe, W. Elger* and *H. Steinbeck*: 18. Mosbacher Koll. d. Ges. f. Biol. Chemie, Springer-Verlag Berlin-Heidelberg-New York p. 218 (1967).

[38] *Neumann, F., W. Elger, R. von Bersword-Wallrabe* and *M. Kramer*: Naunyn-Schmiedeberg Arch. exp. Path. Pharmak. **255**, 221 (1966).

[39] *Neumann, F., W. Elger* and *H. Steinbeck*: Int. J. clin. Pharmacol. **6**, 475 (1968).

[40] *Neumann, F., W. Elger, H. Steinbeck* and *R. von Berswordt-Wallrabe* : 13. Symp. d. Dtsch. Ges. f. Endokrinologie, Springer-Verlag Berlin-Heidelberg-New York p. 78 (1967).

[41] *Neumann, F., K. D. Richter* and *P. Günzel* : Zbl. Vet. Med. **12**, 171 (1965).

[42] *Odell, W. D., G. T. Ross* and *P. L. Rayford:* J. clin. Invest. **46**/2, 248 (1967).

[43] *Ofner, P.:* Vitamines and Hormones **26**, 237 (1968).

[44] *Perklev, T.* and *Y. Gröning* : Acta endocr. (Kbh.) **61**, 449 (1969).

[45] *Peterson, N. T.* jr., *A. R. Midgley,* jr. and *R. B. Jaffe* : J. clin. Endocr. **28**/10, 1473 (1968).

[46] *Scott, W. W.* : In : *Pincus, G.* and *E. P. Vollmer* (ed.) : Acad. Press New York/London p. 179 (1960).

[47] *Scott, W. W.* : Nat. Cancer Inst. Monograph **12**, 111 (1963).

[48] *Suchowski, G.* : Acta endocr. (Kbh.) **27**, 225 (1958).

[49] *Tullner, W. W.* : Nat. Cancer Inst. Monograph **12**, 211 (1963).

[50] *Vogt, H. F.* : Med. Klin. **50**, 1509 (1955).

[51] *Walsh, P. C.* and *R. F. Gittes* : October Meeting of the Amer. Coll. of Surgeons, San Francisco, (submitted for publication, 1969).

[52] *Wollmann, A. L.* and *J. B. Hamilton* : Endocrinology **81**, 350 (1967).

[53] *Wollmann, A. L.* and *J. B. Hamilton* : Endocrinology **81**, 1431 (1967).

[54] *Woodruff, M. W.* and *C. Perez-Mesa* : J. Urol. **88**/2, 273 (1962).

Discussion

J. T. Grayhack: I wish to comment upon Dr. *Salloch's* paper. First of all, in the results he reported, I think it is necessary that he tells us whether he is dealing with the entire prostate weight or with segments of the prostate weight. As you know, various portions of the rat's prostate respond differently to hormonal stimuli. The lateral prostate is stimulated both by oestrogen and prolactin, whereas the central prostate is not stimulated by prolactin. Unless we see the separated results of the response to prolactin between the lateral, dorsal and ventral prostate it is difficult to interpret the data you have presented. Secondly : Do you think that the human has prolactin? There certainly is a lactogen which has been isolated from the placenta. We have utilised it in prostatic studies and have demonstrated that it too is a synergist with androgen in stimulating prostatic growth of the lateral and dorsal rat prostate. But does the human male have a lactogen?

I do not know very much about prolactin in the human male. Dr. *Ilse von Berswordt-Wallrabe* of Göttingen (personal communication) found different results investigating the urine of male students, in some cases there was a prolactin-content as high as in lactating women and in some cases there was a minimum.

The Metabolism of Testosterone in the Prostate

D. C. Williams

The Marie Curie Memorial Foundation, Oxted, Surrey, England

Summary: Hormone therapy, both additive and ablative, is widely used in the control of human prostatic cancer, but the biochemical basis for this treatment is not clear. One of the main problems in the experimental investigation of prostatic cancer is the lack of an animal tumour having properties sufficiently similar to the human disease to give meaningful comparison between them.

It appears likely, however, that the action of testosterone, in the prostate gland of both animals and man, is dependent upon the prior metabolism of the hormone. For this reason a study of the metabolism of testosterone in the normal rat prostate is being undertaken which, it is hoped, will be relevant to our other studies on the culture of human prostatic cancer.

Data is also presented concerning the effect of cyproterone on testosterone metabolism in the normal rat prostate gland. It is suggested that the principal action of cyproterone, under these conditions, is to reduce the cellular level of dihydrotestosterone. The implications of this work as a basis for possible combination therapy are mentioned.

The normal prostate gland is very responsive to androgen stimulation and in a proportion of cases this property is shown in malignant tissues arising from it. This has led to the extensive use of hormone therapy in the treatment of prostatic cancer, but the precise biochemical control mechanism which governs the growth of the prostate gland is still largely unknown.

It is unfortunate that the animal prostate is not a good tool for investigating the human disease since it is difficult to obtain either carcinoma or benign enlargement of the prostate gland in animals. Experimental prostatic carcinomas, which can occasionally be produced experimentally by implantation of carcinogens in the prostate, are usually either hormone insensitive or lose their sensitivity with successive transplantation. These facts severely limit animal experimentation as a method for direct investigation of the human disease. These limitations are further complicated because of differences in response between different species and even, in some cases, different strains of the same species. However, administration of androgens to castrated animals generally results in the rapid growth of the ventral prostate gland together with secretory processes in the epithelial cells, suggesting a common hormonal control mechanism.

Manuscript received: 19 December 1969

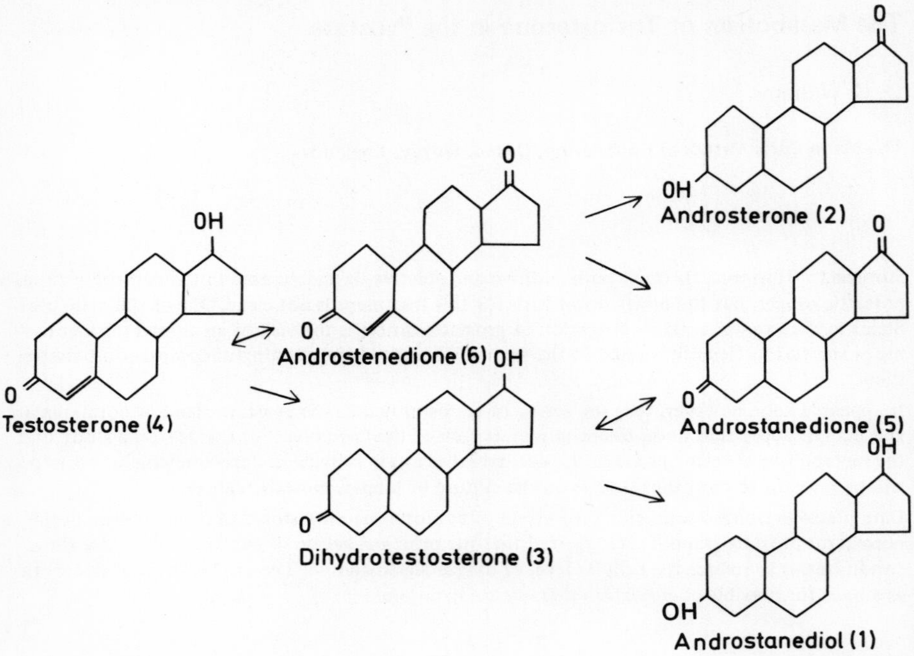

Fig. 1. A simplified scheme for the metabolism of testosterone. The numbers refer to the order of emergence from the vapour phase column shown in Fig. 3.

It is also true that tumours show variations in response between different groups of cells within the tumour so that the biochemical effects observed in tumours are "average" ones for groups of different cells with often wide differences in individual response. Since secondary growths may arise from any particular clone of cells within the primary tumour, it does not necessarily follow that such tumours will be steroid sensitive however successful the primary hormone treatment. The relationship between steroid hormones and prostatic cancer is obscure and there appears to be no direct relationship between steroid hormone levels and clinical state (see [4]).

There is a large body of evidence that the action of testosterone, unlike that of estrogens, is dependent upon the metabolism of the hormone (Fig. 1). It is therefore likely that the metabolism of testosterone is a necessary prerequisite for its hormone action.

[³H] testosterone injected into
intact ligated organ. Incubated
in vitro. Minced and homogenised.

Prostates homogenised, nuclear and
cytoplasmic fractions isolated.
Incubated with [³H] testosterone.

→ Deproteinised with ethanol. ←

— Unlabelled carrier androgens added. —

Extracts evaporated, aqueous
residue partitioned against
ether. Pooled ether fractions
backwashed.

Extracts evaporated and freeze dried.
Residues extracted with ethanol/ether.

Fractions concentrated and applied to
T. L. C. Plates developed in benzene
followed by cyclohexane / acetone.

↓

T. L. C. plates examined under U-V.
Androgen zone removed and eluted
with CHCl₃.

↓

Aliquots taken for separation by
G. L. C. Radioactivity associated
with carrier androgen peaks
determined by scintillation spectrometry.

Fig. 2. The extraction technique used for both *in vitro* and *in vivo* experiments.

Bearing the above limitations in mind, I should like to mention some work which
has been performed by *Belham* and *Neal* [2], working in our laboratories. They
have used, as a model system, the normal ventral prostate gland of the rat, and
have investigated the metabolism of testosterone and the effect of cyproterone
treatment on this metabolism at a subcellular level in this organ. It is hoped that
from studies of this type it will eventually become possible to predict the response
of a particular cell type to a specific steroid at its site of action within the cell.

In this work labelled steroids are administered at a "near physiological" concentration so that their metabolism should bear a relationship to the endogenous compound.

A technique has been evolved in which [³H] testosterone of high specific radioactivity is injected into the prostate, the tissues extracted, and 10 μg each of unlabelled
carrier steroids added to the ethanolic extract. The androgens were then separated
from interfering lipids by thin layer chromatography (Fig. 2). The eluate was applied to a Pye 104 gas chromatograph and separated on a 7ft. 3 % QF₁ column at
215 °C using a flame ionisation detector. The water produced in the detector is collected using a simple modification of the standard apparatus. The condensate was

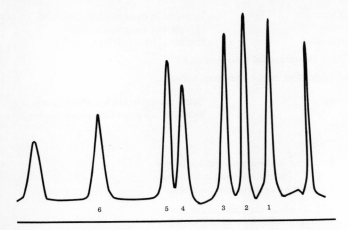

Fig. 3. Vapour phase chromatogram showing the relative positions of testosterone and its metabolites:

1 Androstanediol (5α-androstan-3α, 17β-diol),
2 Androsterone (3α-hydroxy-5α-androstan-17-one),
3 Dihydrotestosterone (17β-hydroxy-5α-androstan-3-one),
4 Testosterone (17β-hydroxy-4-androsten-3-one),
5 Androstanedione (5α-androstan-3, 17-dione),
6 Androstenedione (4-androsten-3, 17-dione).

collected in scintillator and counted in the Beckman apparatus. Radioactivity was recovered to the extent of 81 ± 5 %. During eight replicate experiments, determinations of individual metabolites were within ± 5 %. The separation of the various metabolites which is obtained is shown in Fig. 3.

In the *in vitro* studies ventral prostate glands were excised from adult rats and fractionated in the usual way. Incubations were performed as described by *Bruchovsky* and *Wilson* [3]. Reactions were terminated by chilling to 0 °C. The rate of metabolism of testosterone *in vitro* by the nuclear and cytoplasmic fractions both from untreated tissues and those from cyproterone treated animals is shown in Fig. 4. From these results it appears unlikely that cyproterone exerts its effect by blocking the initial metabolism of testosterone.

The *in vitro* effect of cyproterone on the pattern of testosterone metabolism in both nuclear and cytoplasmic fractions is shown in Fig. 5. An elevation in the amount of labelling associated with dihydrotestosterone in the presence of cyproterone was observed. This figure also shows that dihydrotestosterone and androstanediol are the principle metabolites formed by both the nuclear and cytoplasmic fractions. These findings agree with those of *Bruchovsky* and *Wilson* [3] in the cytoplasmic fraction, but not in the nuclear fraction.

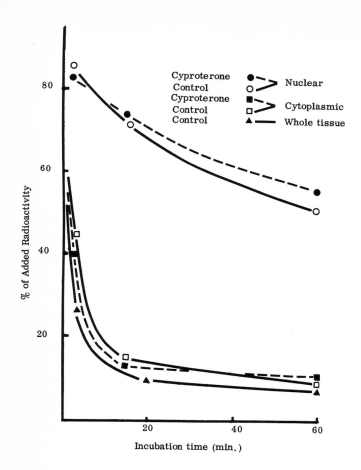

Fig. 4. The disappearance of labelled testosterone during incubations of nuclear and cytoplasmic fractions and whole tissues with and without added cyproterone.

Fig. 6 indicates that, in broad agreement with the findings of *Anderson* and *Liao* [1], dihydrotestosterone is the main testosterone metabolite observed within the nucleus of the prostate cell. In these experiments, animals are treated for a period with cyproterone followed by a single injection of [³H] testosterone and compared with appropriate controls. The similar results obtained in the cytoplasm may relate to the presence of a cytoplasmic androgen receptor which has been indicated by other work in our laboratory.

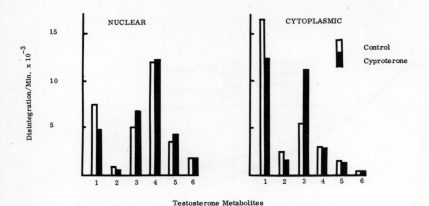

Fig. 5. Radioactive content of testosterone metabolites following *in vitro* incubation of nuclear and cytoplasmic fractions with [³H] testosterone. The numbers of testosterone metabolites refer to the vapour phase chromatogram (Fig. 3).

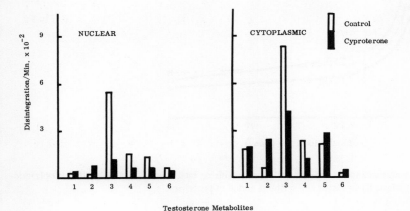

Fig. 6. Radioactive content of testosterone metabolites following *in vivo* administration of [³H] testosterone. The numbers of testosterone metabolites refer to the vapour phase chromatogram (Fig. 3).

Comparison between the last two figures suggest that, whereas androstanediol and dihydrotestosterone are the principle metabolites found *in vitro*, only dihydro-testosterone is found *in vivo*. It appears that either differing metabolic pathways operate or that the androstanediol is not retained by the prostate gland. It would thus appear that selective retention of dihydrotestosterone is more plausible since cyproterone appears to have only a slight effect on testosterone metabolism *in vitro* but caused considerable reduction in the level of labelling observed in dihydrotestosterone *in vivo*. No *in vivo* increase in labelling occurred in the other metabolites examined.

In vitro incubation studies showed that even at the highest concentrations of cyproterone possible, little effect was observed on the metabolism of testosterone by intact prostates, chopped prostatic tissue or sub-cellular fractions. It appeared, therefore, that the anti-androgenic effect could not be due solely to suppressing the formation of an active metabolite. *In vivo* studies, on the other hand, showed that a drastic reduction in the retention of dihydrotestosterone by the prostate was brought about by prior treatment of the animal with cyproterone. Thus, it appeared that a principal action of cyproterone was to reduce the level of dihydrotestosterone in the prostate.

It is probable that cyproterone competes with androgen for receptor sites within the nucleus, probably within the chromatin and especially the euchromatin fractions [5], but there is no such competition between stilbestrol and dihydrotestosterone under similar conditions. It therefore appears likely that anti-androgens of the cyproterone type could be used, with advantage, in conjunction with stilbestrol as a basis for the combination therapy of steroid sensitive tumours.

References

[1]   *Anderson, K. M.* and *Liao, S.* (1968), Nature, **219**, 277.

[2]   *Belham, J. E., Neal, G. E.* and *Williams, D. C.* (1969), Biochim. Biophys. Acta. **187**, 159.

[3]   *Bruchovsky, N.* and *Wilson, J. D.* (1968), J. Biol. Chem., **243**, 2012.

[4]   *Franks, L. M.* (1967), "Recent Research on Prostatic Pathology", in: Pathology Annual, **2**, 76.

[5]   *Mangan, F. R., Neal, G. E.* and *Williams, D. C.* (1968), Arch. Biochem. Biophys., **124**, 27.

Discussion

P. Walsh: Our interest, similar to Dr. *Williams,* is in the mechanism of action of cyproterone acetate. I want to emphasize again that in the prostate the primary metabolic alteration of testosterone is its conversion to dihydrotestosterone by $5-\alpha$ reductase enzymes. Dihydrotestosterone is then bound in the nucleus to the chromatin by an acidic protein. This work has been done by Dr. *Jean Wilson.* With the knowledge that there are two important steps in the intracellular mediation of androgenic action, we looked to see at which step cyproterone acetate acted; whether it blocked the enzymatic conversion of testosterone to dihydrotestosterone or whether it inhibited the binding of dihydrotestosterone to the nuclear protein complex. To test this, we incubated purified prostatic nuclei, the source of the 5-α reductase enzyme, with testosterone-^{3}H and increasing concentrations of cyproterone acetate, Fig. 1. It was clear that with 4000 fold excess of cyproterone acetate, there was no inhibition of conversion of testosterone to dihydrotestosterone. These results were confirmed in *in vivo* studies. Therefore, we felt that the site of inhibition was most likely the binding of dihydrotestosterone in the nucleus. As seen in Fig. 2, we incubated labelled testosterone and dihydrotestosterone with ventral prostate tissue minces and then isolated the nuclei, and determined how much dihydrotestosterone was bound to the nucleus. By adding cyproterone acetate to the incubations, we were able to inhibit the concentration and binding of dihydrotestosterone by up to 6 fold.

In summary, cyproteroneacetate does not effect enzymatic conversion but we feel that it acts by competitively inhibiting dihydrotestosterone binding to the nucleus presumably by competitive inhibition of binding. We feel that these steps are important not only for the study of the mechanism of the action of anti-androgens but now give us a new biochemical approach to the understanding of the loss of hormonal dependence of carcinoma of the prostate.

Fig. 1. Influence of CA on *in vitro* conversion of T-^{3}H to DHT-^{3}H by prostatic nuclei.

Concentration of CA	% T Converted to DHT	% T Converted to A	Total % T Converted to DHT + A
None	75.2	13.7	88.9
2.4×10^{-8}M	77.4	14.8	92.2
2.4×10^{-7}M	78.2	13.8	92.0
2.4×10^{-6}M	75.2	14.7	89.0
1.2×10^{-5}M	79.9	4.6	84.5

Fig. 2. Inhibition of nuclear uptake *in vitro* by CA.

Concentration of CA	Cytosol cpm/gm	Nuclei total cpm/mg DNA	Nuclei bound cpm/mg DNA
Testosterone-1,2-^{3}H 1.2×10^6 cpm			
None	151,240	3470	1270
3.4×10^{-8}M	143,720	3375	920
3.4×10^{-7}M	161,290	1465	410
Dihydrotestosterone-1,2-^{3}H 1.8×10^6 cpm			
None	41,240	6630	2360
3.4×10^{-8}M	36,990	3870	1350
3.4×10^{-7}M	44,260	1610	455

Pharmacological Aspects on the Treatment of Prostatic Carcinoma with Stilbestrol Diphosphate

N. Brock

Pharmacological Department of the Asta-Werke AG, Chemical Factory, Brackwede, Germany

Summary: The superior therapeutic effect of high doses of stilbestrol diphosphate (STDP) in human prostatic cancer cannot be explained by an indirect effect via the pituitary. In addition a direct effect of the liberated stilbestrol on prostatic cancer tissue is involved. This concept is supported by the clinical experience according to which STDP is only effective in the high dosage range which leads to stilbestrol concentrations in prostatic tissue 100 times those seen in other tissues. With regard to the mechanism of action the following points are discussed:

(1) STDP is split by prostatic phosphatase to form free stilbestrol.
(2) After adequate doses of STDP (single dose > 500 mg) cumulation of free stilbestrol in the prostate or in prostatic carcinoma.
(3) Stilbestrol does not only exert a cytostatic effect on the isolated tissue of the prostate (tissue sections or tissue cultures), but also on other cells, i. e., it has direct cellular effects.
(4) There is no parallelism between the antigonadotrophic and estrogenic effects of STDP and its therapeutic action in prostatic carcinoma.
(5) The absence of side effects particularly on the breasts and the intense therapeutic effect on prostatic carcinoma speak in favour of the drug's local, i. e., tumour-specific action.
(6) Even in estrogen-resistant patients and also after surgical castration STDP still produces therapeutic benefit in prostatic carcinoma.

I have been asked to speak as a pharmacologist about the treatment of prostatic carcinoma with stilbestrol diphosphate. Ten years ago this invitation would have given me great pleasure, but the passionate discussions about the mechanism of action of this preparation date back as far as ten years and new experimental results have been scarce since then. As yet there is no experimental model available for prostatic carcinoma, which would allow elucidation of all questions at issue. Thus I fear that the essential pharmacological points of view about which I am going to report, are already known to you. Therefore I can put it briefly and restrict my contribution to the essential point, which centres particularly around the discussion of clinical experience which has repeatedly been reported in world scientific literature until quite recently.

Manuscript received: 13. November 1969.

C. H. Huggins [25, 26] was the first to prove prostatic carcinoma and other hormone-dependent tumours to be subject to the same hormonal actions as normal tissue, both with regard to proliferation and biochemical functions. Based on this knowledge *Huggins* introduced orchectomy and estrogen therapy as "antiandrogenic" measures into the treatment of prostatic carcinoma. The estrogen "diethyl stilbestrol" was the first synthetic agent which allowed to improve disseminated carcinoma in man.

Nowadays the mechanism of action of estrogen treatment is generally interpreted as follows [24]:

Prostatic carcinoma shows properties of the normal epithelial cell of the prostate in that its growth also depends on the blood androgen level. Low androgen concentrations produce a slight, high androgen concentrations an increased growth of normal, and almost invariably also of degenerated prostatic epithelium. Via the diencephalic PSC the estrogens reduce the gonadotrophic activity of the anterior pituitary and thus inhibit the formation of androgens in the testicles. Thus an essential growth-promoting agent is eliminated for both the prostate as a secondary sex organ and for prostatic carcinoma so that hormonal castration results.

According to general experience the favourable effect of the estrogens is restricted to the duration of treatment. However, the necessary prolonged maintenance treatment with estrogens is often associated with untoward side effects such as mammary reactions *(gynaecomastia)* and sooner or later resistance to treatment develops. Therefore improvement of this type of treatment appeared to be desirable.

Such an advance was made by *Druckrey* and *Raabe* [16] who in 1952 suggested the use of stilbestrol diphosphate [1]) in the treatment of prostatic carcinoma for the following reasons:

(1) In contrast to free stilbestrol, its diphosphate is readily soluble in water and high doses can easily be administered by the i.v. or oral routes.
(2) Local and general tolerance is excellent.
(3) STDP is split by the acid prostatic phosphatase which liberates active stilbestrol.
(4) In addition to its estrogenic effect, stilbestrol itself possesses pronounced cytostatic properties.

Since the carcinomatous prostatic tissue and its metastases usually have a very high phosphatase activity, the drug is supposed to be preferably split *loco dolenti*, its readily soluble transport form being thus converted into the slightly soluble "active form" which then cumulates and acts within the prostatic tissue, whereas the unchanged STDP is readily eliminated again. In addition to the drug's well known effect on the diencephalo-pituitary system this new concept also implies a direct effect of the liberated stilbestrol on the cancer cells of the prostate.

---

[1]) Honvan [®], Asta-Werke AG, Chemical Factory, Brackwede

„Transport form" $Na\ HO_3P - O - \bigcirc - C = C - \bigcirc - O - PO_3HNa$

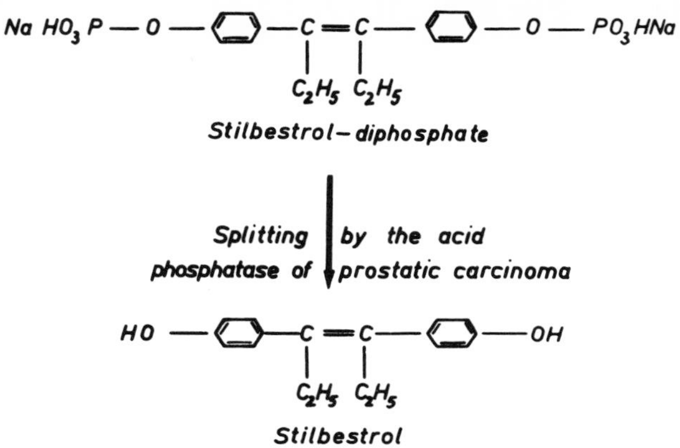

$C_2H_5\ C_2H_5$

Stilbestrol–diphosphate

Splitting | by the acid
phosphatase of | prostatic carcinoma

„Active form" $HO - \bigcirc - C = C - \bigcirc - OH$

$C_2H_5\ C_2H_5$

Fig. 1

Stilbestrol

As confirmed by numerous German and foreign publications, STDP has proved to be of particular therapeutic benefit [6]. *Gaca* et al. [19] of the Surgical Unit of Freiburg University Hospital, who in 1968 published their results obtained in 176 sufferers from prostatic carcinoma during a period of 13 years, report a 5-years' survival rate of 42 %. Even patients who no longer responded to the usual treatment with free estrogens, showed a definite improvement in one third of the cases which shows STDP to be doubtless superior to free estrogens [30, 36].

The above theoretical concept aroused a good deal of controversy in the early sixties [7, 9, 10, 11, 12, 23]. Whereas its advantage of solubility in water, its local and systemic tolerance and great therapeutic potency were recognised, the following points of its mechanism of action were doubted:

(1) cleavage *in vivo,*
(2) cumulation of the liberated estrogen in the prostatic cancer cells and
(3) its direct cytostatic effect.

(1): The cleavage of STDP by acid prostatic phosphatase has been adequately proved [4, 16]. *Arnold* and *Klose* [2] studied the conversion of STDP into free stilbestrol and demonstrated stilbestrolmonophosphate to be formed as an intermediate. *Hohlweg* and *Groot-Wassink* [24] have proved this conversion also to occur *in vivo.* In the rabbit they showed 64 % of the administered STDP dose to be eliminated in the form of glucuronate, which can however only be formed after previous cleavage of the phosphate. The equipotent estrogenic effects of STDP and free stilbestrol observed by *Druckrey* and *Kaiser* [14] in the vaginal smears of spayed rats does not necessarily imply that the ester itself exerts an estrogenic effect, but it may readily be attributed to the liberation of stilbestrol from STDP, the more so as the estrogenically active dose is very low (e.g., about o.5 μg in the rat) and the high phosphatase activity in blood and tissue has proved to ensure the drug's rapid cleavage *in vivo.*

| Dose Stilbestrol-diphosphate (mg) | Concentration of free Stilbestrol | | Accumulation in Prostate |
	Fat or Muscle (μg)	Prostate (μg)	
50	<0,025	<0,025	–
125	<0,025	0,025	slight
500	<0,025	0,25	10 X
1000	0,25	25	100 X
2000	0,25	25	100 X

Fig. 2. Concentration of free estrogen in 10 g tissue 1 h after i.v. infusion of stilbestrol-diphosphate − in dependency on dosage − in patients suffering from prostatic carcinoma (according to [35]).

(2): In spite of the well proven cleavage, various authors doubted the cumulation of the liberated stilbestrol in the prostate [17, 24]. From the outset cumulation appeared only probable if the concentration of stilbestrol liberated in the prostate surpassed the solubility threshold. The solubility of stilbestrol in human serum is 100 mg/l, thus exceeding by far the value expected from its slight solubility in water. Thus cumulation of the liberated stilbestrol in the prostate can only be expected with very high doses of STDP after which the stilbestrol concentration within the tissue lies above the critical solubility limit. The correctness of this view was confirmed by measurements made by *Segal, Marberger* and *Flocks* [35] in man. Prior to surgery they treated sufferers from prostatic carcinoma or prostatic hypertrophy with various doses of STDP and subsequently they compared the resulting concentrations of free stilbestrol in the prostatic, adipose and muscular tissues (Fig. 2). After administration of small doses ($\leq$ 125 mg) of STDP, localisation of stilbestrol in prostatic tissue was not detectable. However, between the 1st and 8th hour after injection of 500 mg the concentration was about 10 times that of other tissues, and after 1000 and 2000 mg it was even 100 times that found in muscular and adipose tissues. Thus the possibility of obtaining considerable concentrations by massive-dose treatment has been proved. In his studies with ^{14}C-labelled stilbestrol diphosphate *Ghaleb* [20] obtained principally the same reults, which he summarises as follows:

"With the phosphate ester there was considerable localisation in the prostate, mainly in the form of free stilbestrol. This probably results from hydrolysis of the ester by the acid phosphatase in the prostate. With free stilbestrol there was no such localisation".

(3): Even the direct effect of STDP or free stilbestrol on prostatic carcinoma cells was subject to a good deal of controversy. The opponents of this concept [23, 24] argued that STDP would only act as an estrogen and that its therapeutic effect would only be based on the inhibition of the gonadotrophic pituitary function and the resulting reduction of testicular secretion of androgens. However, the drug's biological effect is also directly exerted on the peripheral pituitary-dependent organs and tissues. Thus *Dirscherl* and *Brever* [8] verified the direct effect of estrogens on the prostate by measuring the intracellular metabolism of isolated tissue, and it was confirmed even more convincingly by *Lasnitzki* [27] and *Franks* [18] in prostatic tissue cultures. In addition many investigations were able to prove the cytostatic effect of stilbestrol (but not of STDP) on other types of highly proliferative tissues or cells such as the fertilised egg of the sea urchin [13], paramaecia [5] and tissue cultures [28, 31] and finally even in malignant tumours of man and animals [29, 34]. According to these results stilbestrol is generally considered to be a highly active mitotic poison. In this connection a paper recently published by *Harper* et al. [21] is of interest. These authors found diethylstilbestrol and even its diphosphate to inhibit the DNA polymerase of the prostate *in vitro* in as low concentrations as of 10 nmol. This doubtlessly implies a direct effect on mitosis. On the other hand, the introduction of so-called pituitary blocking agents such as 4-hydroxypropiophenone [32] has been disappointing in prostatic cancer. In a paper on the treatment of hormone-dependent tumours, *Boyland* [3] argues that even the therapeutic effect of free stilbestrol in prostatic carcinoma cannot be explained by its antigonadotrophic effect alone, but it must equally be attributed to a direct effect on the tumour cells.

The difference between the drug's estrogenic effect and its direct effect on prostatic carcinoma tissue is best demonstrated by the clinical results. Whereas free estrogens invariably produce more or less marked enlargement of the breasts, such a side effect is rare and less pronounced after STDP inspite of the latter's potent antitumour action in prostatic carcinoma. In this connection *Purvis* and *Denstedt* [33] speak of the "perplexing question why no side effects are observed upon administration of STDP". This shows STDP to exert a more "directed" organo-specific effect which is also verified by the fact that prostatic carcinomas resistant to free estrogens still respond to high doses of STDP and often continue to respond for many years. Moreover, the fact that even after surgical castration STDP still allows therapeutic benefit to be obtained in prostatic carcinoma, speaks against the assumption that the antitumour action is due to its antigonadotrophic effect alone.

Thus I think an approach based on the "as-well-as" law in biological behaviour to be more in conformity with the scientific findings than the restriction to the "either-or" rule. However, for the direct inhibitory action of liberated stilbestrol to become effective on prostatic tissue, adequate concentration *loco dolenti* is absolutely essential. With the usual form of stilbestrol pellet implantation, the threshold concentration is certainly not reached, but the concentration of 25 μg in 10 g of prostatic tissue (i.e., 100 times that found in other tissues, reported by *Segal* et al. [35], will suffice to produce direct therapeutic effects of several hours' duration. In the fertilised egg of the sea urchin much lower concentrations produced intense antimitotic effects, after only a few minutes' action.

The mechanism of action of any drug invariably represents an intricate problem. For STDP and even for the free estrogens, it has not yet been fully elucidated. Some of the pending questions can only be answered if an adequate model for human prostatic cancer will be available. The working hypothesis "transport form/active form" — whether recognised or not — has also proved of value in other fields of cancer research, e.g., in general cancer chemotherapy with the cyclic N-mustard phosphamide esters [1] and in the carcinogenic action of nitrosamines [15]. As shown by *W. Heubner* [22] in his paper on "Creative Ideas and Chance in Drug Research", it can still be considered as a true creative idea.

References

[1]   *Arnold, H., Bourseaux, F.* and *Brock, N.:* Naturwissenschaften **45,** 64 (1958).

[2]   *Arnold, H.* and *Klose, H.:* Arzneimittel-Forsch. **7,** 471 (1957).

[3]   *Boyland, E.:* Symposium on Cancer Chemother., Tokyo (1960).

[4]   *Brandes, D.* and *Bourne, G. H.:* Lancet S. 481 (1955).

[5]   *Brock, N.:* Zweites Freiburger Symposion über Grundlagen und Praxis chemischer Tumorbehandlung, 17.–19.7.1953, S. 266, Springer-Verlag (1954).

[6]   *Brock, N.:* Z. Krebsforsch. **62,** 9 (1957).

[7]   *Brock, N.:* 7. Symposion d. Dtsch. Ges. f. Endokrinol. Homburg (1960).

[8]   *Dirscherl, W.* and *Brever, H.:* Z. Krebsforsch. **59,** 253 (1953).

[9]   *Dörner, G.* and *Zabel, H.:* Zbl. Gyn. **81,** 1788 (1959).

[10] *Dörner, G.* and *Knappe, G.:* Klin. Wschr. **38,** 67 (1960).

[11] *Druckrey, H.* and *Brock, N.:* Münch. Med. Wschr. **102,** 1626 (1960).

[12] *Druckrey, H.* and *Brock, N.:* Münch. Med. Wschr. **103,** 777 (1961).

[13] *Druckrey, H., Danneberg, P.* and *Schmähl, D.:* Naturwissenschaften **39,** 381 (1952).

[14] *Druckrey, H.* and *Kaiser, K.:* Dtsch. Med. **81,** 1084 (1956).

[15] *Druckrey, H., Preussmann, R., Ivankovic, S.* and *Schmähl, D.:* Z. Krebsforsch. **69,** 103 (1967).

[16] *Druckrey, H.* and *Raabe, S.:* Klin. Wschr. **30,** 882 (1952).

[17] *Ferguson, J. D.:* Brit. J. Urol. **30,** 397 (1958).

[18] *Franks, L. M.:* Brit. J. Cancer **13,** 59 (1959).

[19] *Gaca, A., Köhnlein, H. E.* and *Köttgen, H.:* Med. Welt **19**, 961 (1968).

[20] *Ghaleb, H.:* Brit. Emp. Cancer Campaign. Ann. Rep.: **37**, 145 (1959).

[21] *Harper, M. E., Pierrepoint, C. G.* and *Griffiths, K.:* Biochem. J. **114**, 58 (1969).

[22] *Heubner, W.:* Pharmaz. Z. **101**, 378 (1956).

[23] *Hohlweg, W.* and *Dörner, G.:* Münch. Med. Wschr. **102**, 2603 (1960).

[24] *Hohlweg, W.* and *Groot-Wassink, K. A.:* Dtsch. Gesundh.-Wesen **14**, 152 (1959).

[25] *Huggins, C.:* Klin. Wschr. **36**, 1102 (1958).

[26] *Huggins, C.* and *Hodges, C. V.:* Cancer Res. **1**, 293 (1941).

[27] *Lasnitzki, J.:* Cancer Res. **14**, 632 (1954).

[28] *Lettre, H.:* Hoppe-Seyler's Z. Physiol. Chem. **278**, 201 (1943).

[29] *Mayer, S.* and *Morton, M. E.:* Experientia **12**, 322 (1956).

[30] *McKinnon, K. J., Nearing, T. N.* and *Carruthers, N. C.:* Canad. med. Ass. J. **77**, 1009 (1957).

[31] *Moellendorf, W. v.:* Klin. Wschr. **18**, 1098 (1939).

[32] *Perrault, M.:* Presse méd. **59**, 1010 (1950).

[33] *Purvis, J. L.* and *Denstedt, O. F.:* Dep. of Biochemistry McGill University of Montreal. personal communication (1956).

[34] *Schmähl, D.:* Arzneimittel-Forsch. **4**, 481 (1954).

[35] *Segal, S. J., Marberger, R.* and *Flocks, R. H.:* J. Urol. **81**, 474 (1959).

[36] *Wilmanns, H.:* Medizinische, **1**, 17 (1954).

Discussion

R. H. Flocks: I want to say a word or two with regard to Prof. *Brock's* talk on diethyl stilboestrol diphosphate. He mentioned our original work by *Marberger* and *Segal* which had to do with the presence of the concentration of the stilboestrol in the prostate. The time interval was not emphasised. The stilboestrol stayed in the prostate approx. 8 hours following the intravenous infusion and then the concentration went down. In a subsequent article by *Harris, Hummel* and others in our laboratory, we showed with tag material that the concentration was 100 times higher in the prostate than it was in the tissue adjacent to the prostate in the human, we did not test the kidney, lung or bone marrow in the human because these were patients in whom we did not feel it wise to do this. In the animal, however, the concentration in the liver, kidney, lung and bone marrow of this compound was in the order of about 1000 times higher than it was in the prostate, and much higher than it was in the blood or in the fat, and in the fibrous and muscular tissue adjacent to the prostate. This would seem to indicate that certainly the stilboestrol itself is not a cytotoxic substance, certainly as far as the liver, kidney, lung and bone marrow were concerned and therefore does not act in a cytotoxic manner.

J. T. Grayhack: I would like to comment on Prof. *Brock's* paper. The basic assumption that we have made is that data with regard to normal prostate has had value in studying and treating prostatic carcinoma. We have attempted on several occasions to demonstrate that there was a local inhibitory effect of oestrogen on prostatic growth. We put pellets of various oestrogens directly into the ventral prostate of the rat and have demonstrated no inhibition of weight nor of anything else. We placed pellets of oestrogen alone and oestrogen and androgens combined into dog's prostates and studied the surrounding area histologically. The only thing we have found was an overgrowth of prostatic epithelium. While it is true that the character of the prostatic epithelium has been changed markedly in fact we have seen no evidence of a cytotoxic effect from the local oestrogen. We would like you to comment on that if you would.

N. Brock: Dr. *Flocks,* when administering stilboestrol diphosphate in high doses, you obtained an accumulation of free, non-phosphorylated stilboestrol in lungs and kidneys, but no functional change or cell damages in these organs. Dr. *Bagshaw* made the same question as to the direct effect of the drug. I feel that there is a distinct difference between bringing a drug either into contact with normal cells or with cells having a high rate of proliferation as it is the case with tumour cells. *Dirscherl* and *Brever, Franks, Lasnitzki, Moellendorf* and *Druckrey* did also use in their studies cell cultures containing highly proliferative cells, and *Schmähl* studied the effect of stilboestrol in the Walker carcinosarcoma of the rat. It is not realistic to transfer results obtained with one type of cells directly to other cells. The same applies to direct conclusions obtained in one species of animals to either other species or the human being. The problem of the selective cancerotoxic activity is well known to me from studies with cyclophosphamide and its activation, where 90 % of activation occurs in the liver, the highly active primary metabolite concentrating in liver, lungs and kidneys. However, we did not detect any biological effect in these organs, e.g.,the liver function was never disturbed, but the metabolite has been traced in cancer tissue and in all sites of high cell proliferation.

One factor is the permeation rate of different compounds in various cell types. We know that the cancer cell has other permeation possibilities than the normal cells. I am certain that the antimitotic activity of the two phenolic groups of stilboestrol cannot be disproved. Studies with the egg of the sea urchin and with cell cultures definitely confirmed the strong antimitotic activity of stilboestrol. The direct antimitotic effect is already released by very small quantities of e. g. 0.5 μg/ml, which is indeed a very low concentration. Cell division is completely stopped. The mechanism of action, however, is still unknown, and much work remains to be done in this field.

H. Marberger: I would like to comment on Prof. *Brock's* paper. I must say that our group along with our former boss Dr. *Flocks* disagree on the 3 points you have said to be settled today : First on the place of cleavage and hydrolisation of stilboestrol disphosphate. Secondly we disagree on the concentration. A concentration of 100 times is a misleading figure because this is in comparison with fat,and fat has a very low uptake. It is very much higher in other tissues, in the liver, in the kidney, in the lung, in the testicles and in other places which have fast growing tissues. Thirdly on the mode of action. We tried several compounds. We tried to analyse them and track them by acid phosphatase and it never went as we thought it would go. The hydrolisation occurred in other places. The idea behind the theory is as follows. – You inject water-soluble oestrogens. They arrive at the prostate. They are split in the prostate and the stable compound stays there. The stable cytostatic compound stays there and acts as a cytostatic agent. But this theory is not true. Neither does stilboestrol nor do other cytotoxic compounds which have been made stay in the prostate. So as Dr. *Flocks* mentioned, after 8 hours the stilboestrol disappears and within 10 hours most of it was gone and after 48 hours it was completely gone. From the compound we made and labelled we had very little activity after 10 hours and we had none after 48 hours. So cytotoxic effects must be much less than other effects that we see in patients, because in the patients we have very, very good therapeutic effects from water soluble stilboestrols. We still use it and we like the drug very much and we have quite a series of patients, but we do believe that the mode of action is on another basis. Maybe the dosage plays a role, different pharmacological effects resulting from high blood levels over a short period, compared with low dosage and low blood levels or compared with long continuous blood levels.

N. Brock: It is generally known that establishing the true mode of action of specific drugs involves many problems. A real distinction should be made between well established facts on one hand and so-called research hypotheses on the other. Therefore, I want to summarize the following facts:

1. It is well proved that stilboestrol diphosphate is freely soluble in water and is split in the prostatic gland by the action of the prostatic phosphatases. However, this applies only to the human prostate, the prostatic cancer in particular, but not to animals (the only exception being the dog). That is why, experimental results obtained with animals, cannot be regarded as valid in man.

2. The liberated stilboestrol is sparingly soluble in water. This leads to accumulation of stilboestrol in the normal human prostate and in prostatic cancer tissue. This only occurs, provided very high doses are given, exceeding the soluble portion of stilboestrol. Depending upon the actual concentration and the solubility in body fluids, a constant elimination occurs, so that the initial high concentration is only of shorter duration.

3. A direct cytostatic effect is only possible during cell division. For example the mitotic rate in the liver is about 1 : 20 000 whereas it is by hundred times higher in cancer tissue. The cytostatic action of stilboestrol diphosphate has been proved in various cell types.

4. The therepeutic activity of stilboestrol diphosphate against prostatic carcinoma has also been pointed out by *Marberger* to be very good, although this action cannot fully be explained by a pure hormonal effect. We agree with *Marberger's* opinion that dosage not only plays a certain rôle but must be regarded as decisive. This applies in particular to the first dose.

5. Nevertheless, the elucidation of the mode of action of this drug remains an interesting problem. This is demonstrated by the fact that stilboestrol monophosphate is, in contrast to the diphosphate, rather toxic, but less effective in the therapeutic sense. This difference also shows that the results obtained by *Hummel, Harris, Marberger* and *Flocks* with diphenylphosphamid-phenyl-phosphoric acid do not permit to draw any definite conclusions with regard to stilboestrol diphosphate.

6. The high therapeutic action of stilboestrol diphosphate has also been confirmed by *Ghaleb's* study. He also found a much higher concentration of liberated stilboestrol in the human prostate than in muscle tissue, although the dose of 270 mg he used was too low.

J. D. Fergusson: I would like to ask Prof. *Brock* if he has any current explanation for the pain which patients get in the back following the infusion of phosphorylated oestrogens. If he believes that this is due to the concentration in the prostate can he explain why, when we give this infusion to women, they also get pain in the same place.

N. Brock: At present, there is no explanation available.

W. W. Scott: In the early 40's while I was working with Dr. *Huggins* we determined the acid phosphatase in the urine. If one measures the acid phosphatase activity of the young male it is roughly about 100 units per 24 hours. In the young female, about 100 units per 24 hours. These are King Armstrong units. Now the adult male puts out about 600 units per 24 hours, K. A., but the figure for the adult female is not 100 but 400 units. So we conclude there are glands along the urethra between the bladder and the meatus which are producing acid phosphatase and if the *prostate* is able to hydrolyse this compound, why can't these glands?

Pathology of Cancer of Prostate

F. K. Mostofi

The Armed Forces Institute of Pathology and the Veterans Administration Special Reference Laboratory for Anatomic Pathology at the AFIP, Washington, D. C. 20305, USA

Summary: The pathological criteria for diagnosis of carcinoma of the prostate, the differential diagnosis and the factors of importance in prognosis have been briefly reviewed. An attempt has been made to establish an objective parhological basis for grading and prognostication in cancers of the prostate.

1. Introduction

It is a high honor for me to be invited to this great city and to participate in this important conference. My first visit to Berlin was 38 years ago — early November, when I stopped in Berlin for 3 days on the way from Iran to the United States for my education. Many important events have happened since then and although this is the first trip to Berlin since then, Berlin has remained in my memory as the first European capital. I am also happy to be back in Germany where I have so many good friends of many years, both among the urologists and the pathologists.

The comments that I shall make on the pathology of carcinoma of the prostate are based on the experience that I have gained from 21 years at the U. S. Armed Forces Institute of Pathology in Washington. During that period I have seen over 12, 000 cases of prostatic cancers. Included in this group is the pathological material from over 2,000 biopsies and 250 total prostatectomies of the Veterans Administration Urological Cooperative Research Group study. As Dr. *Mellinger* will mention in detail, total prostatectomy was done in Stages I and II prostates. Stage I denoted prostatic carcinomas that were incidental pathologic findings in a transurethral resection for a clinically benign hyperplastic prostate, and Stage II denoted those that had a nodule in the prostate and the tumor was entirely confined to the prostate. My report, based on the studies of these 12,000 cases, will be general comments not in any way intended as an analysis of the series.

Manuscript received: 13 November 1969

2. Criteria for pathological diagnosis of carcinoma of the prostate

Carcinoma of prostate presents a wide range of histological patterns unequalled by any other malignant epithelial tumor (Figs. 1–17) and poses many problems in diagnosis.

Cellular anaplasia, invasion and metastases are the three classical pathological criteria for the diagnosis of carcinoma, but these are often missing in prostatic carcinoma and we must add to these criteria disturbances of normal architecture.

2.1. Anaplasia (Fig. 1–4)

In anaplastic carcinoma usually the nuclei are large, but there is considerable variation in size and shape of nuclei; they have an irregularly thickened nuclear membrane, uneven distribution of chromatin, one or two large rod shaped nucleoli and a large single intranuclear vacuole. The cytoplasm is either granular or vacuolated; mitosis and giant cells are present. The cells vary a great deal in size and shape, they may form glands of varying sizes and types or they may occur as solid sheets, columns or individual cells.

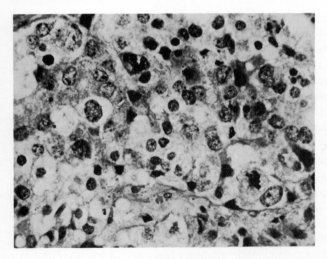

Fig. 1. Anaplastic carcinoma (Grade III). Note the variation in size, shape and staining of nuclei. One definite mitotic figure is seen. AFIP Neg. 70-3952 X 450.

Such evidences of anaplasia are well recognized and when present readily lead to the diagnosis of carcinoma of prostate. Regrettably, however, many of the tumors especially in the early stage, show little or no anaplasia. Many of the carcinomas have fairly uniform small nuclei with a delicate membrane and a fine network of evenly distributed chromatin. Mitosis and giant cells are rare. While careful examination may show some variation in staining, size and shape of nuclei, and an abnormal nuclear-cytoplasmic ratio, nevertheless, many pathologists experience difficulty in diagnosing carcinoma.

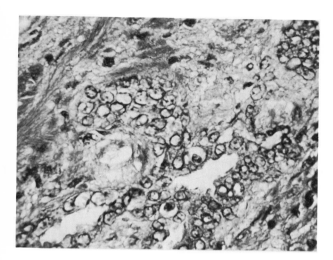

Fig. 2. Anaplastic carcinoma (Grade III). The nuclei show variation in size and shape, and contain a single large vacuole. AFIP Neg. 70-3946 X 520.

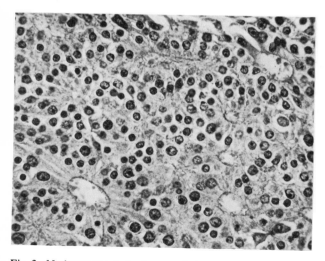

Fig. 3. Moderate anaplasia. Some variation in size and staining of nuclei. AFIP Neg. 70-3936 X 450.

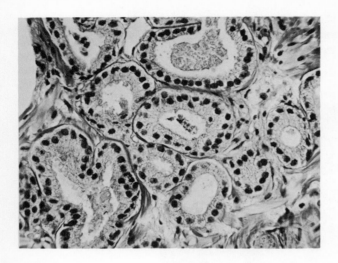

Fig. 4. Slight anaplasia (Grade I). Most of the nuclei are of uniform size, shape and staining. AFIP Neg. 70-3945 ✕ 350.

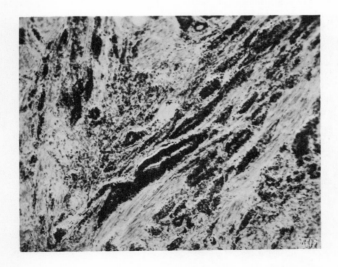

Fig. 5. Carcinoma of prostate. The acid phosphatase stain shows many dark granules in the epithelial cells. This is very helpful in diagnosis of carcinoma of prostate. AFIP Neg. 52-3133 ✕ 115

2.2. Invasion (Fig. 6—8)

In such cases we must search for evidence of invasion — of the stroma, of the perineural spaces, of the capsule, of the seminal vesicles or of the adjacent organs. In biopsies, especially when the tumor is confined to the prostate, we must depend on invasion of the stroma and the perineural spaces.

In 1952 [1], I emphasized invasion of the stroma, as a criterion for diagnosing carcinoma but until recently there has been considerable discussion on whether, in fact, a basement membrane is present around the prostatic acini. The existence of a basement membrane has now been demonstrated by the electron microscope [2].

Invasion of the intraprostatic perineural spaces occurs in about 90 % of the prostatic carcinomas and is an unequivocal pathological evidence for the diagnosis of carcinoma. While the finding of perineural invasion is diagnostic of carcinoma of prostate, many biopsies do not show this and we must look for other evidences of malignancy.

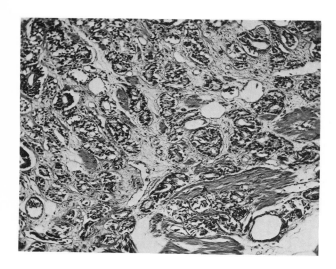

Fig. 6. Carcinoma of prostate. The tumor infiltrates the stroma. No basement membrane is seen in A. AFIP Neg. 70-82062 X 130.

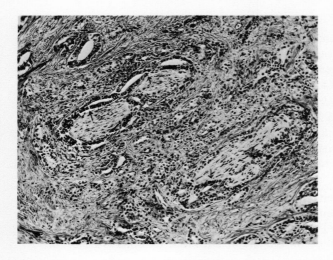

Fig. 7. Carcinoma of prostate. The tumor infiltrates the perincural spaces (arrows). AFIP Neg. 70-2068 ✕ 130.

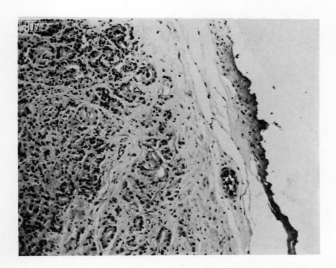

Fig. 8. Carcinoma of prostate. The tumor invades the subserosa. AFIP Neg. 52-5180 ✕ 125.

2.3. Extension and metastases

Extension beyond the confines of the prostate to the capsule, to the seminal vesicles, to the serosa and to the adjacent organs or metastasis as evidenced clinically by elevated acid phosphatase, positive x-ray, or positive bone marrow or supraclavicular or other lymph node biopsies would certainly confirm the diagnosis of carcinoma of prostate but these are absent in the earliest stages.

2.4. Disturbances of architecture (Fig. 9–17)

Some years ago [1], I emphasized that where anaplasia and invasion are equivocal and extension and metastases are absent, disturbances of architecture, as compared to the normal or hyperplastic prostates, are of greatest help: haphazard distribution of acini, many small acini, microacini, acini that are closely packed, acini that are devoid of convolutions, acini that occur inside other acini and sheets of cells with no acini are among the features that help us in diagnosing carcinoma.

2.5. Histochemical aids

The presence of colloid substance, and the demonstration of positive acid phosphatase in histological sections are also often helpful (Fig. 5).

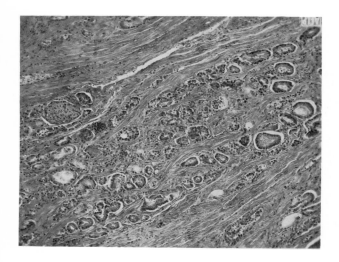

Fig. 9. An incidental carcinoma. Note the wide range in the size of the acini from very small to large ones, distributed haphazardly in the stroma. AFIP 488132 X 180.

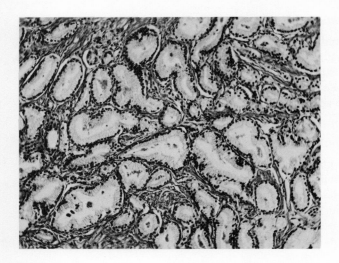

Fig. 10. Carcinoma of prostate. The tumor forms large glands without convolutions. There is a single layer of nuclei. No convolutions are seen. The basement membrane is often absent. AFIP Neg. 70-2112 ✕ 130.

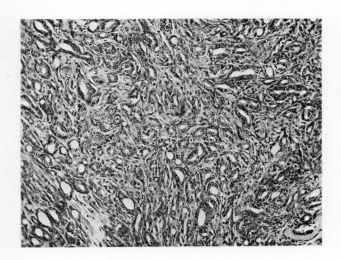

Fig. 11. Carcinoma of prostate. The tumor forms many small glands which are closely packed. Some stroma is seen in between acini. AFIP Neg. 70-2134 ✕ 130.

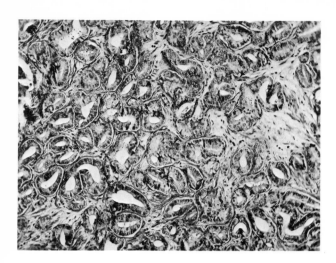

Fig. 12. Carcinoma of prostate. The tumor forms large acini without any convolutions. The acini are arranged haphazardly. AFIP Neg. 70-2136 X 130.

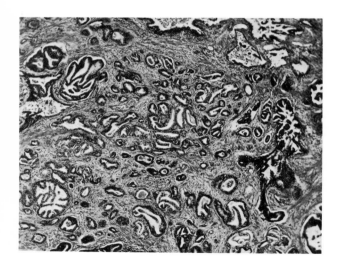

Fig. 13. Carcinoma of prostate. The tumor forms glands of varying sizes with some small, others that are irregular and still others that form glands in glands. There is haphazard distribution of glands. AFIP 591506 X 60.

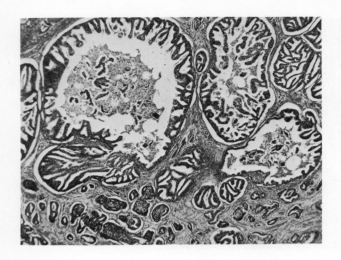

Fig. 14. Carcinoma of prostate. The tumor forms glands of varying sizes ranging from small to large. Several large glands are seen with papillation and glands in glands. AFIP 591506 × 60.

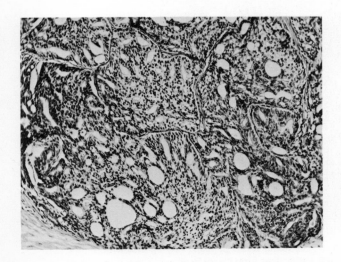

Fig. 15. Carcinoma of prostate. The tumor forms glands in glands. AFIP Neg. 70-2060 × 145.

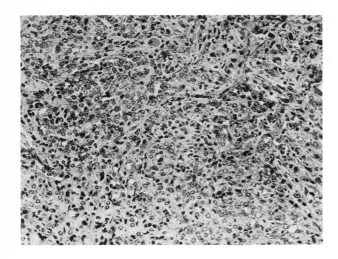

Fig. 16. Carcinoma of prostate. The tumor forms solid sheets with little or no intervening stroma. AFIP 488132 ✕ 180.

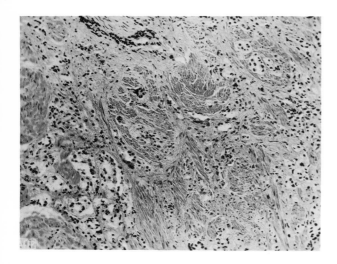

Fig. 17. Carcinoma of prostate. There is overgrowth of stroma with only scattered tumor cells – some forming glands – and resulting in a scirrhous carcinoma. AFIP 63204 ✕ 125.

3. Lesions that simulate carcinoma of prostate (Fig. 18—24)

Calculi, atrophy of the prostate, infarction and granulomatous prostatitis may mislead the urological surgeon to diagnose carcinoma. This is particularly true for granulomatous prostatitis which may involve the capsule. It must be emphasized that any hard nodule in the prostate must be regarded as carcinoma unless proved otherwise; on the other hand a total prostatectomy on such cases is not justified without microscopic or other confirmation. In seeking such confirmation caution must be exercised in interpreting an elevated acid phosphatase because, while the enzyme is elevated in 60 % of patients with prostatic carcinoma and 80 % of those with bony metastasis, there may be other causes of elevated acid phosphatase: digital manipulation, recent or old infarction, *Paget's* or other bone disease, *Gauchers*, multiple myeloma and hyperparathyroidism. Secondly, it is important to determine not only total serum acid phosphatase but the prostatic fraction as well [3].

Microscopically, typical and atypical hyperplasia (Fig. 18), secondary hyperplasia (Fig. 19), metaplasia (Fig. 20 and 21), atrophy (Fig. 22), seminal vesicles (Fig. 23) and granulomatous prostatitis (Fig. 24) are not infrequently misdiagnosed as carcinoma by the pathologist. Time does not permit me to detail the characteristic features of each of these but these have been discussed elsewhere [3, 4, 5].

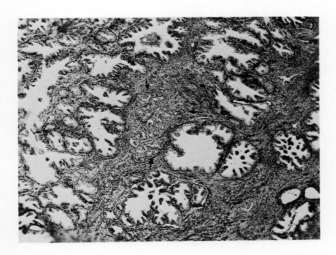

Fig. 18. Atypical hyperplasia. Excessive infolding of hyperplastic epithelium is seen. Note a small area of carcinoma with microacini (arrows). AFIP 584064 ✕ 50.

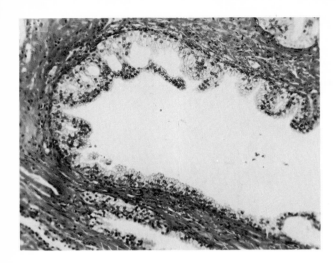

Fig. 19. Secondary hyperplasia. A dilated erstwhile gland is partly lined by hyperplastic epithelium which froms structures resembling glands in glands. Compare to Figures 10 and 11. AFIP Neg. 52-5124 X 145.

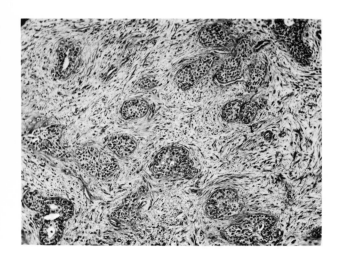

Fig. 20. Transitional cell metaplasia. Nests of transitional cells are seen surrounded by newly formed exuberant fibrous stroma representing healed infarct. The focus simulates carcinoma but the cells are regular and display no anaplasia. AFIP Neg. 69-9740 X 100.

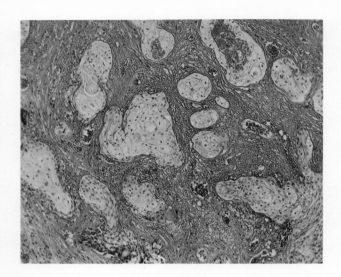

Fig. 21. Sqamous metaplasia. Nests of well differentiated mature squamous cells are seen in an area of recent infarction. These foci are often mistaken for squamous carcinoma but no evidence of malignancy is seen. AFIP 140643 X 90.

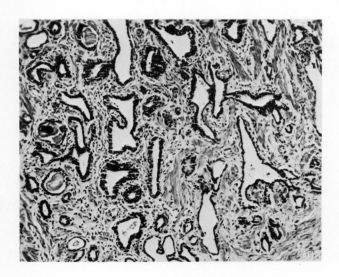

Fig. 22. Atrophy of prostate. The glands are lined by cells with dark staining nuclei. These simulate carcinoma. The acini are devoid of convolutions and at times collapsed. The nodular architecture is maintained. AFIP Neg. 52-2783 X 115.

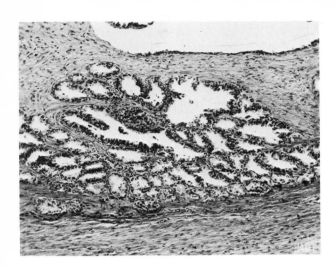

Fig. 23. A section of seminal vesicle. The back to back arrangement of ducts, some of which are lined by hyperchromatic nuclei resembles carcinoma. Note the organoid pattern and intraluminal and superficial position of the hyperchromatic cells. AFIP Neg. 52-3126 X 75

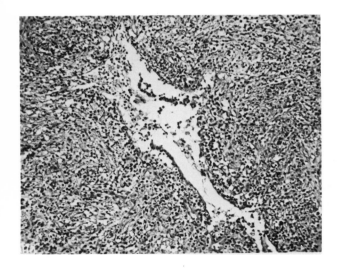

Fig. 24. Granulomatous prostatitis. The prostate is infiltrated with many small cells, many of which have vacuolated cytoplasm. The infiltrating cells resemble carcinoma but note the relationship to a duct whose epithelial lining is in part desquamated. AFIP Neg. 52-3993 X 130.

4. Grading of carcinoma of prostate

Pathologists like to grade the tumors as an expression of the prognosis of the tumor. This has been difficult if not impossible to do in carcinoma of the prostate.

a) Carcinoma of the prostate is a slow growing tumor and even after metastases have occurred, with proper therapy and sometimes even without therapy, the patient may live for many years.

b) While the anaplastic pleomorphic undifferentiated carcinomas (Fig. 1,2) and the well differentiated carcinomas (Fig. 5, 6) are readily recognizable as bad (Grade III) and good (I) tumors, respectively, and these are fairly well correlated with prognosis, many tumors fall in between and these as well as some of the Grades I and III carcinomas have an unpredictable behavior.

c) Many carcinomas show an amazing range of morphological patterns which tend to prevent quantitation. In recent years, *Gleason* [5, 6] has designed a method to circumvent this. He recognizes a primary and a secondary pattern and, in each, one or more of five or more patterns from the most differentiated to the most undifferentiated.

d) The major difficulty with all efforts to grade carcinoma of prostate has been that the criteria for anaplasia and differentiation have not been clearly defined, and much of the categorization has been subjective. We have proposed an objective and systematic method based on the status of three elements in the prostate — the glands, the epithelial cells and the stroma. We separate tumors that form glands (Fig. 5—11) from those that do not (Fig. 12): those that form glands are further subdivided to those with normal glands (Fig. 10, 12, 13), those with large glands (Fig. 14), those with small glands (Fig. 9, 11), and those with cribriform pattern (Fig. 15). The epithelium can show no anaplasia (Fig. 4), some anaplasia (Fig. 3), or considerable anaplasia (Fig. 1, 2). The tumor stroma can be of normal amount (Fig. 11, 13, 15), increased (Fig. 17), decreased or absent (Fig. 11, 15, 16).

5. Location of the tumor and its significance in the choice of biopsy for diagnosis of carcinoma

The posterior lobe has been considered for many years as the site of origin of most carcinomas of prostate. This was confirmed by our study, but many foci were also found in the lateral lobes. It is of interest to note that in two instances the tumor was confined to the anterior area and in several others it had extended to this region. Since ordinarily no glands are encountered in the anterior lobe of human male prostates, these probably represented extensions of the lateral lobes.

I prefer to separate the prostate into peripheral and central, as has been done by *Adrion* [8] and more recently by *Franks* [9]. We found that in 45 % the tumor was confined to the periphery, in 54 % it was both peripheral and central; and in only two cases did we find carcinoma centrally without any obvious peripheral tumor. We saw several instances where a large well encapsulated hyperplastic nodule was the cause of obstruction and tended to compress the carcinoma to the periphery.

The fact that most of the early carcinomas of prostate are at the periphery has an important relationship to the choice of the method of biopsy in patients suspected of carcinoma. In a recent study we selected 308 patients on whom we had both transurethral resection (TUR) and needle biopsies (NB) [10]. We divided these into two groups: The unequivocally advanced carcinoma by which we meant those in which carcinoma comprised more than 25 % of the available tissues examined by the microscope. There were 200 in this group, 195 were positive by both methods (NB and TUR). In the second group we placed all those in which carcinoma comprised less than 25 % of the entire available tissue. We classified these as early or intermediate. We had 108 in this group. Both NB and TUR were positive in 58, whereas TUR was positive in only 76 while NB was positive in 96.

Hudson and *Stout* [11] have shown that TUR yields positive results in only 50 % of clinically suspected cases. Thus it appears that perineal or transrectal, open or needle biopsy or retropubic biopsy is more reliable for the diagnosis of carcinoma of prostate than TUR, because the earliest carcinomas are located at the periphery. Transurethral resection must be primarily for the relief of obstruction and not for diagnosis of carcinoma.

6. Comparison of clinical and pathological findings

The study of surgically removed total prostates has enabled us to compare the urologist's findings on rectal examination (always recorded on special forms as part of the study protocol) with the pathological findings on examination of the tissue [12]. Clinically, most of the prostates either had no nodule or a single nodule, while pathologically we found that 84 % had either multiple foci or extensive carcinoma — only 16 % had a single focus. In about 25 % we found penetration of the capsule and/or extension to the seminal vesicles by our microscopic studies where it had not been detected on rectal examination by the urologist. Of tumors which both clinically and pathologically were confined to a single focus, 32 % showed invasion of the capsule and 5 % penetration of the capsule. In tumors with multiple foci the figures were 36 and 15 %, and for extensive diffuse tumors, the figures were 33 and 58 %, respectively. Thus in 76 % we found, through careful pathological examination of the specimen, more tumor than the urologist suspected from his careful rectal examination.

7. Factors that may affect the prognosis

Three factors may affect the biological behavior of a tumor:

a) response of the host,
b) reaction of the physician, and
c) the basic potentialities of the neoplasm.

Little is known about the first; a discussion of the second may be properly left to the urological surgeons. I have discussed the potentialities of the tumor elsewhere [3, 5] but they may be summarized here.

While it is generally agreed that prostatic carcinomas in older patients (78 or over) show infrequent metastasis, data relating to tumors in the young are somewhat contradictory. *Tjaden, Culp* and *Flocks* [13] observed that many young patients are in advanced stages (but an occasional one may live a long time with little or no treatment) while *Byar* and *Mostofi* [14] have found that patients less than 50, if diagnosed early, do better than older patients. Patients with symptoms for 12 months seem to do better than those with shorter or longer periods. Patients with blood group AB fare better. Patients with hypertension or urinary tract infection are said to have better prognosis than those with patent upper urinary tract. Incidental, focal, and small carcinomas, and those that are totally removed have a better prognosis than clinically manifest or diffuse carcinomas, or those that are large or incompletely removed. Carcinomas that are confined to the prostate, those that have not metastasized, those whose metastases are osteoblastic, those which metastasize to soft tissue and the lungs, those that have normal or low total and prostatic acid phosphatase do better than those with extension, with metastasis to bone, with osteolytic metastasis or with consistently elevated phosphatases.

Patients with diploid and tetraploid tumor chromosomes have better prognosis than those with haploid or hexaploid.

In a recent yet unpublished study, Dr. *Byar* and I [12] have demonstrated that certain pathological findings indicate better prognosis: tumors located at the periphery compared to those both centrally and peripherally; those with single foci compared to those with multiple foci, those without microscopic involvement of the capsule and/or the seminal vesicles compared to those with microscopic penetration of the capsule or the seminal vesicles.

Perineural invasion has no appreciable significance on prognosis.

Pathological grading, especially when combined with clinical staging may have prognostic value. A number of studies have shown that very few patients with anaplastic and poorly differentiated tumors survive more than 5 years and *Gleason* and his associates [6, 7], have reported favorable results with their method of grading when combined with staging. Our own studies have shown that better prognosis may be expected for tumors that form glands, those in which the glands are regular, those in which the epithelial cells are of about normal size, and without nuclear anaplasia, those in which the glands are back to back, or the stroma is essentially normal. Work on establishing a simple reproducible method of grading is continuing with the hope that a single element can be found on which the pathologist can prognosticate with reliability.

Acknowledgement: This study was supported in part by the Veterans Administration Cooperative Urological Research Group.

References

[1] *Mostofi, F. K.:* Criteria for pathological diagnosis of carcinoma of prostate. Proc. Second Nat. Ca. Conf., 332, 1952.

[2] *Mao, P., Nakao, K.* and *Angrist, A.:* Human prostatic carcinoma: An electron microscopic study. Cancer Res., **26**, 955, 1966.

[3] *Mostofi, F. K.:* Carcinoma of the Prostate. In: Modern Trends in Urology, edited by *Riches, Sir Eric.* London, Butterworth & Co., 1969.

[4] *Mostofi, F. K.:* Hyperplasia of the Prostate. In: Textbook of Urology, edited by *Campbell, M. F.,* and *Harrison, J. H.* Philadelphia, W. B. Saunders Co., 1970.

[5] *Mostofi, F. K.* and *Price, E. B.* Jr.: Tumors of the Male Genital System (Fascicle). Atlas of Tumor Pathology. Second Series, Armed Forces Institute of Pathology, Washington, D. C. (In Prep.)

[6] *Gleason, D. F.:* Classification of prostatic carcinoma. Cancer Chemother. Rep., **50**, 125, 1966.

[7] *Mellinger, G. T., Gleason, D. F.* and *Bailar, J.,* III.: The histology and prognosis of prostatic cancer. J. Urol., **97**, 331, 1967.

[8] *Adrion, W.:* Ein Beitrag zur Aetologie der Prostatahypertropathic. Beitr Path Anat **70**, 179, 1922.

[9] *Franks, L. M.:* Benign nodular hyperplasia of prostate. A review. Ann. Roy. Coll. Surg. Engl., **14**, 92, 1954.

[10] *Purser, B. N., Robinson, B. C.* and *Mostofi, F. K.:* Comparison of needle biopsy and transurethral resection biopsy in the diagnosis of carcinoma of the prostate. J. Urol., **98**, 224, 1967.

[11] *Hudson, P. B.* and *Stout, A. P.:* Prostatic Carcinoma XVI. Comparison of physical examination and biopsy for detection of curable lesions. New York J. Med., **66**, 351, 1966.

[12] *Byar, D. P.* and *Mostofi, F. K.:* Carcinoma of the prostate: Prognostic evaluation of certain pathological features in 208 radical prostatectomies. (In preparation).

[13] *Tjaden, H. B., Culp, D. A.* and *Flocks, R. B.:* Clinical adenocarcinoma of the prostate in patients under 50 years of age. J. Urol., **93**, 618, 1965.

[14] *Byar, D. P. and Mostofi, F. K.:* Cancer of the prostate in men less than 50 years old: An analysis of 51 cases. J. Urol., 102, 726, 1969.

Discussion

W. E. Goodwin: Prof. *Alken* wanted me to ask Dr. *Mostofi:* "How can you determine the potential malignancy of a prostate cancer? " In other words, what guidelines can you give us, (apart from your study of 300 cases) now or for the future, as to which way the studies should be directed to determine potential malignancy?

F. K. Mostofi: I think this point about malignant potential of a carcinoma of prostate is very difficult. We can separate the anaplastic Grade III carcinomas. That leaves us a large number of Grade I (good) and II (intermediate) tumors. Dr. *Belt,* Mr. *Fergusson,* Dr. *Jewett,* Dr. *Flocks* and Dr. *Mellinger's* work have given us some guide lines: When the tumor is small, confined to the prostate, when it is completely removed at first operation with surrounding normal tissue, when it is entirely inside the capsule, when it is a single nodule or when it is incidental carcinoma the prognosis is good. Some years ago in a report from Dr. *Flocks'* department (*Tjaden, H. B., Culp, D. A.,* and *Flocks, R. H.:* Clinical adenoca in patients under 50 years of age. J. Urol. 93, 618, 1965) it was shown that young patients with carcinoma of the prostate do poorly. We have recently studied 51 patients less than 50 years of age and find that in this group the survival was better than in a comparable older age group. However, our patients were U. S. Army personnel in whom the lesions were picked up on routine annual physical examination including rectal examination, which is mandatory. High acid phosphatase before operation, persistently elevated acid phosphatase or recurrence of elevated acid phosphatase after it has dropped post therapy are bad signals! As far as the tumor itself is concerned we must admit that at the present we do not have a reliable prognostic criterion on individual tumors. Some of the apparently good tumors will metastasize and kill, some of the bad tumors will survive for many years.

W. E. Goodwin: Second question: What is the frequency of occurrence of a unilocular cancer, that is just localised in one place versus the frequency of multiple cancers in the prostate.

F. K. Mostofi: My experience has been that it is really extremely rare to have a single focus of carcinoma. Now it is true that when you do a rectal examination, you feel one nodule, but often there are many more. I am sorry that I cannot give the specific figures – but I think the majority of carcinomas (as I see it in the total prostate) have more than one nodule of carcinoma.

C. E. Alken: Rectal examination in Germany is not done by practitioners, and very seldom by highly specialised people in other disciplines. So it happens that most of all prostatic cancers we see, are in the 2nd or 3rd stage.

This is the reason, why we have no broad experience in radical prostatectomy. I would like to know if the perineal approach is better than the retro-pubic approach.

R. H. Flocks: I want to first expand a little bit on the discussion which Dr. *Mostofi* delivered on Pathology of prostatic cancer. I want to emphasise that he found that in his studies only 1 % of the lesions were in the central part of the gland. The rest were in the peripheral or showed microscopic extension outside the capsule. This is extremely important if we are considering at all the aggressive ablation and destruction of a local lesion. Secondly, I want to emphasise that in approx. 25 % of the patients who have prostatic lesions which are relatively small but probably do show extraprostatic extension, that exploration of the pelvis will show a definite involvement of the regional lymph nodes. In larger lesions this percentage increases. So that, as we have reported previously and others have reported, the percentage may go as high as 87 %, even though there is no clinical evidence of bone metastasis or elevation of the serum acid phosphatase. Thirdly, I want to emphasise that in about 10 % of the patients even small lesions which seem to be operable on rectal examination, and this is really confirmed by the study by

Dr. *Ormond Culp* of the Mayo Clinic recently, about 10 % will show osteoblastic changes on strontium isotope studies, which can not be seen on the ordinary X-ray films and without elevation of the serum acid phosphatase. So we have here something which needs to be considered very seriously in our attempts, if we are to attempt aggressive attack upon the local lesion. We need to consider the presence or absence, the possibility of regional lymph node metastasis and of vascular metastasis. I was very much interested in the figure that Dr. *Mostofi* showed which had to do with the presence of a bunch of tumour cells in the middle of a vein.

M. A. Bagshaw: I would like to ask Dr. *Mostofi* to enlarge a little bit on the evidence that perineural spaces are not lymphatics and further to ask whether or not if they are not lymphatics they may be in some way continuous with the lymphatic system.

F. K. Mostofi: Rodin and his associates (*Rodin, A. E., Larson, D. L.,* and *Roberts, D. K.*: Nature of the perineural spaces invaded by prostatic carcinoma. Cancer **20**, 1772, 1967) have shown that these spaces are not lymphatics but simply perineural spaces. They communicate with the perineural spaces in the capsule and in periprostatic tissue but whether they also communicate with lymphatic spaces I do not know but I doubt it. I might mention that there is some question about the existence of a lymphatic system in the prostate but it seems doubtful that an organ like prostate would have no lymphatics.

W. W. Scott: Dr. *Mostofi* had asked me to answer a question which relates to grading of tumours. In our series of radical perineal prostratectomies at Johns Hopkins (these data can be found in the January issue of the JAMA for 1969) it seemed quite clear that the grade of the tumour at least as we determined it histologically affected the prognosis. There were no 15 years' survivorship in patients with 1 cm nodules or less, subjected to total perineal prostatectomy, who had poorly differentiated carcinoma. All were well differentiated carcinomas. Now many of these patients with well differentiated, small nodular carcinoma where the carcinoma was confined to the substance of the prostate gland histologically had invasion of the peri neural spaces. Finally there were no 15 years'survivorship in the nodule group when the cancer had spread to the perivesicular fascia.

H. Marberger: You told me that the carcinoma of the prostate is multilocal and the various foci differ in grade and stage.
What does this mean in regard to exact histological grading? How big a piece do you have to take? Do you think that the information you get from a needle biopsy is a really good information?

F. K. Mostofi: Grading is difficult in prostatic carcinomas. This stems from the fact that carcinoma of the prostate varies considerably from one area to another. In grading a tumor there should be consistency on the same slide by the examiner himself and he should be able to define the criteria in such a manner that others can duplicate his grading.
In grading prostatectomy specimens I found that I could not be consistent with my own grading unless I graded exactly the same microscopic area. With needle biopsies it is a little easier but is still quite difficult. Dr. *Gleason* of Veterans Administration Hospital in Minneapolis, USA, has devised a method which he believes helps him in this work. He recognizes a primary and a secondary pattern and in each separates the tumor into one of 9 categories with 1 representing the incidental tumors and 9 the anaplastic. He then adds the results of patterns 1 and 2 with the stage of the tumor and can provide a "prognostic index". Dr. *Gleason's* classification is still in preliminary trial stages and it has not been possible to reproduce it. Quantitation is difficult if not impossible for prostatectomy specimens but for needle biopsy it is easier since the amount of tissue is so small. The important thing is to clearly establish and define the criteria for anaplasia and differentiation and make it objective as we are trying to do, then grading can be reproduced; otherwise it is all subjective.

H. Marberger: But how big? What is the information you need from a needle biopsy as far as grading is concerned? Would you think that this is good information?

F. K. Mostofi: The information obtained from needle biopsy is fairly good when it is positive. In fact I would much rather grade a needle biopsy than a prostatectomy specimen. The correlation is very good. The fact that grading is possible and is reliable on a tiny bit of tissue removed by needle biopsy is quite interesting. It may well be that the tissue removed by needle is from the oldest portion of the tumor since it is in the peripheral portion where we know carcinoma of prostate originates.

C. E. Alken: I understood from Dr. *Mostofi* that 84 % are multi-locular carcinomas. So if we do a needle biopsy and get a negative result, how many cylinders must be taken?

W. E. Goodwin: Well, we usually take at least three from different areas in the prostate. Always from the suspected area but also from multiple areas. Some years ago Dr. *Kaufman* did a very careful study in which he compared needle biopsy, rectal palpation and open biopsy. He made some observations about the numbers of positive cylinders in relation to the number of biopsies. Dr. *Kaufman*, when you do a needle biopsy, how many cores do you take?

J. J. Kaufman: A minimum of 3. We have done needle biopsies for some 10 years at the UCLA and feel that it is a very important procedure. We think it is very important to use good needles. In our hands, the Vim Silvermann needle is the best, but it must be a relatively new one, not used more than 6−10 times. As soon as the prongs become separated it no longer functions adequately to get good tissue. I do not champion the trans-perineal needle biopsy more than the trans-rectal. It depends upon your experience and upon your particular preference, but I think that you must take multiple cylinders. Now in answer to Dr. *Goodwin's* question: A small nodule is full of pitfalls and errors. The cytology, in our hands − except for extensive carcinoma of the prostate − was also full of false negatives. But the needle biopsy was the best, short of an open perineal biopsy, which we still feel is the definitive way to make a histological diagnosis of prostatic cancer.

W. E. Goodwin: Another one in the audience can comment on this because he is the inventor of a special kind of a needle for biopsy of the prostate: Dr. *Ralph Veenema:*

R. J. Veenema: We have used since 1950 a needle which has a cup on the end which can be palpated in the perineum to increase accuracy. As Dr. *Kaufman* said, the individual must get used to a type of needle and thus increase his accuracy. The suspicious area in the prostate is best biopsied at the first pass of the needle. On the average, we also, do 3 biopsies from the area of clinical involvement.

F. Balogh: I would like to ask Dr. *Mostofi:* Did you examine the prostatic cancer tissue after oestrogen treatment and orchiectomy and what were your findings?

F. K. Mostofi: The effect of orchiectomy on the prostate and on the carcinoma is atrophy. Orchiectomy does not destroy the tumor. It removes a considerable amount of the androgenic stimulus which is useful if and as long as the tumor is hormone responsive.
Oestrogens bring about marked atrophy of the prostate, squamous metaplasia of the ducts and acini and increased fibrous tissue. The effect is both on the epithelium and the stroma. Not all carcinomas of the prostate are responsive to oestrogens but those that are, show vacuolization of cytoplasm, pyknosis of nuclei, disintegration of cell membrane and fragmentation of nuclei. Stromal hyalinization and fibrosis is sometimes quite prominent. We have seen a case in which there was a distinct sarcomatous element and it was suggested that this may have been oestrogen induced.

A. Kelâmi: I would like to show you a new technic to diagnose prostatic cancer. It was first inaugurated in 1960 by *Franzén* in Stockholm, Sweden. We have used this technic for 1 1/2 years, and we have had very good results. The main advantage of this technic is that you can perform it without any anaesthesia, even local anaesthesia is not necessary. It can be performed as an office procedure, and can be repeated at any time.

The instrument is a vacuum pistol with three needles. The needles have a diameter of 0.7 mm. We always do three aspirations. The whole procedure is called "fine needle aspiration biopsy".

The patients do not feel any pain at all, and as I said before, the biopsy can be repeated as often as necessary. We observed no complications so far — neither bleedings nor infections.

The aspirated material is smeared onto slides and sent to the cytologist for evaluation.

R. T. Turner-Warwick: I would like to discuss briefly the diagnosis of the early prostatic tumour. All discussions in its management presuppose that we have an accurate diagnosis. A needle biopsy must always risk spread of the tumour in the tract, some probably more than others, and some routes more than others. Nevertheless, if you are dealing with the treatment of a potential carcinoma in situ, you must bear in mind that you are converting it from a carcinoma in situ, by the process of needle biopsy, and if you make the analogy with a nodule in the thyroid, you would not dream of putting a needle into it; you would make a proper excision. Nevertheless, I want to show you, very briefly, a biopsy needle which we have used, in my clinic, for some 15 years. It is slightly different from the available needles. It produces a very sharp, clean-cut tissue, which is so undistorted, that it can be used for electron microscopy studies.

It is a trephine needle, mounted on a syringe. The needle here is hollow, and there is a stilette which occludes the needle, so that when you withdraw the piston, the stilette is withdrawn causing suction and an empty needle.

It is *not* an aspiration needle. It will produce a clear cut specimen of tissue. I usually prefer the perineal route for this procedure.

G. Jönsson: As to the question of the fine needle biopsy, we have used the method in my clinic for more than 4 years, and we have done several hundred cytological investigations. I must say that we have found a very good correlation between the cytological and histological findings. So I can recommend the method, but you must have a good cytologist, for only then you can get a good answer. It is also of value, if you wish to do repeated biopsies when following up a patient. You can do it in "out patients", without pain or anaesthesia.

Hormonal dependency of prostatic carcinoma in tissue culture

W. E. Goodwin: I would like to ask Prof. *Lars Röhl* to speak to us. He has done some interesting experiments with tissue culture.

L. Röhl: Ten years ago I did a study on hormonal dependency of prostatic carcinoma in the tissue culture, to investigate the prostatic hormone dependency at the cellular level, for there are many contradictory things in prostatic carcinoma, we see latent carcinoma with a very heterologous histologic character, some patients are doing very well with the antiandrogenic therapy, others do not. Therefore I think it is very important that we try to improve the present methods of investigating the biological properties of the prostatic tumour. This was the first publication of a human prostatic carcinoma highly differentiated, and we could show that it was stimulated to proliferate by androsterone in vitro.

The same culture we stained for acid phosphatases and we saw the epithelial cells loaded with acid phosphatases.

With androsterone stimulation there was high proliferation in this tumour.

We cultured about 50 tumours, and we could use about 8 of them. We were sure that these were prostatic malignant epithelia. Their hormone dependency seemed to be coupled to the highly differentiated carcinoma cells, which might explain why the cells, when they go through a very proliferative phase, drop their androgen dependency.

We know that a tumour in its developmental history drops certain characteristics and gains others. This might be an explanation why you *had to* know which type of population you are actually dealing with when you see the tumour.

The first example shows a tumour under anti-androgenic treatment. You have a regression of the androgen dependent cells. Clinically the tumour gets smaller, and you end up with a tumour which contains non-androgen cells. You have a clinical tumour control. It is not an absolute tumour control, but clinically the tumour has not manifested itself.

The 2nd type: When you give your anti-androgenic therapy in this type, you can get away the androgen-dependent cell population. There will be temporary regression, but then these "non-androgen" cells dominate the tumour, it grows again and your anti-androgenic therapy has no effect.

That is the type of patient we see daily. The 3rd type is the tumour that is completely composed of "non-androgen" sensitive cells, and of course your anti-androgen measures have no effect at all. This is the tumour that grows and sooner or later kills your patient. I think that the application of the progression theory can give us important information about which lines we have to renew in the therapy and how it should be done to get a more effective dose. It is not the androgen dependent cell fraction in the tumor, which is the problem in treatment. We can treat it but the "non-androgen" population is the difficulty. The way better therapy will have to go is in the direction of a fractionated therapy. We must try to get some possibility of valuing the biological state of the actual cell population, as for instance to analyse them in tissue culture. I think it is very important, with all respect to the rats and dogs, that we concentrate all our strength on investigating human material, because with these basic thoughts, I think one can understand and explain a lot of the contradictions in our discussions about prostatic cancer. It is not actually possible to discuss prostatic cancer before we know what sort of tumour we are actually dealing with.

N. Brock: I have a question for Prof. *Röhl.* You say we have 2 kinds of cells — hormone dependent and non-hormone dependent cells, and that the relation between these 2 kinds changes with the course of time . . . . Now my question: everyone of us knows patients who are controlled by treatment with oestrogens and with stilboestrol diphosphate for 5, 6, 7, 10 years. What has happened to these 2 kinds of cells now? I imagine that if I can inhibit the hormone dependent cells, why do the non-hormone cells not multiply and why don't these cells kill the patient much earlier? If we transplant a cell from the human or animal body into a cell culture, we are not always sure that it is the same type of cell we have in the body. There is always a trend that specific cells change to unspecific cells. I do not think that cells in cultures behave in just the same way as cells in the human body.

The Incidence of Cardiovascular Complications in Prostatic Cancer

G. T. Mellinger and C. Blackard

Veterans Administration Hospital, Kansas City, Missouri, USA
Veterans Administration Hospital, Minneapolis, Minnesota, USA

Summary: (1) Prostatic cancer patients treated with a 5.0 mg daily dose of diethylstilbestrol have an increased incidence of fatal and non-fatal myocardial infarction, congestive heart failure associated with ischemic heart disease, and cerebrovascular accidents when compared to placebo in all stages. These complications of estrogen therapy are most likely due to an increased incidence of thromboembolism.

(2) Early endocrine treatment of patients with asymptomatic Stage III carcinoma is not indicated. Therapy with diethylstilbestrol, 5.0 mg daily, does not increase the survival of Stage III patients when compared to placebo. The decrease in cancer mortality associated with the 5.0 mg dose of diethylstilbestrol is more than compensated for by an increase in deaths from cardiovascular causes.

(3) Endocrine therapy should be started early only in Stage IV patients where its main value is to relieve such cancer symptoms as bone pain. When estrogen is the preferred endocrine treatment, it would seem wise to administer diethylstilbestrol in only a 1.0 mg dose. This is especially true if electrocardiographic abnormalities are present before treatment, even though there may be no previous history of cardiovascular disease.

An increase in cardiovascular deaths in patients receiving 5.0 mg of diethylstilbestrol daily for prostatic carcinoma has been shown by the Veterans Administration Cooperative Urological Research Group. [1, 2] One criticism of this study is that older men, in whom prostatic carcinoma is found most often, already have a high incidence of cardiovascular problems. *Hanash* and his associates [3] concluded from an examinations of necropsy material that the degree of coronary and aortic atherosclerosis was no worse in patients who had been taking estrogen than in those who had not. They attributed the increased mortality to fatal congestive heart failure, but failed to consider the additional effects of thromboembolism associated with the administration of estrogen [4]. Females taking oral contraceptives have shown an increase in fatal and non-fatal thromboembolism without an apparent increase in atherosclerosis [5].

In its original publications, the Veterans Administration Cooperative Urological Research Group did not take into consideration the cardiovascular status of patients prior to receiving diethylstilbestrol. The Group's earlier papers also did not take into consideration those patients on study who suffered a myocardial infarction,

Manuscript received: 13 November 1969

cerebrovascular accident, congestive heart failure, or any other cardiovascular problem, and yet survived. Now we wish to discuss the incidence and degree of cardiovascular disease in both living and dead prostatic cancer patients, both before and
after the initiation of therapy with diethylstilbestrol.

1. Material and methods

Between March 1, 1960, and February 28, 1969, Stage III and Stage IV prostatic
carcinomas were diagnosed by needle biopsy or transurethral resection in 673 patients
admitted to the Minneapolis Veterans Administration Hospital. 182 patients were
rejected from the study because they had received previous endocrine therapy, had
a second malignancy other than cancer of the skin or lip, were in physical condition
so poor that any of the study treatments might endanger life, had a psychosis, or
lived so far from the hospital that they could not be followed. The other 491 patients with either Stage III or Stage IV prostatic carcinoma were placed on study.
These patients were randomly assigned either to estrogen alone, orchiectomy with
placebo, orchiectomy with estrogen, or placebo alone. The estrogen and the placebo
were double-blinded. Up until two years ago, a 5.0 mg daily dose of diethylstilbestrol
was used exclusively. However, a second study has been instituted during the past
two years, in which the 5.0 mg dosage has been randomly assigned along with placebo,
0.2 mg, or 1.0 mg daily dosage of stilbestrol. Because of the small number of patients
and the short period of follow-up in those receiving 0.2 mg or 1.0 mg of stilbestrol
daily, 54 men in these two groups have been eliminated from analysis, leaving 437
patients to be considered. Men receiving placebo and 5.0 mg of stilbestrol in the
second study have been added to those in the first study. Because bilateral orchiectomy could conceivably influence susceptibility to cardiovascular disease, an additional
204 patients treated by either orchiectomy alone or orchiectomy combined with
estrogen were eliminated from analysis. This left 114 patients who received placebo
alone and 119 who received as their primary therapy diethylstilbestrol alone, in a
5.0 mg daily dose. As of May 31, 1969, there was 100 % follow-up of these 233
patients.

The primary treatment according to the stage of the prostatic carcinoma is shown
in Figure 1. 9 of 148 Stage III patients (6 %) and 19 of 85 Stage IV patients (22 %)
required a change in treatment, either because their clinical condition was deteriorat-
ing or because they could not tolerate the primary drug.

The average age or mean age of patients in each category of treatment was 70.3
years for those receiving placebo and 70.7 years for those taking 5.0 mg of stilbestrol
daily. Patients placed on 5.0 mg of stilbestrol were followed for an average of 34.4
months as opposed to the group on placebo, which was followed for an average of
31.9 months.

Primary Treatment	Number of Patients in Stage	
	III	IV
Placebo	72	42
Diethylstilbestrol 5.0 mg daily	76	43
Total	148	85

Fig. 1. Primary treatment according to the stage of the prostatic cancer.

2. Survival rates and causes of death

Survival rates were determined for Stage III and Stage IV patients receiving placebo or 5.0 mg of stilbestrol daily, employing the acturial or life-table method described by *Cutler* [6]. Analysis of survival data has been done in terms of the primary treatment to which the patient was assigned.

56 of 148 patients in Stage III and 63 of 85 patients in Stage IV died. Survival curves for Stage III and Stage IV patients, comparing placebo to 5.0 mg of stilbestrol, are shown in Figures 2 and 3. There was no difference in survival at any follow-up period between placebo and estrogen-treated patients in either Stage III or Stage IV.

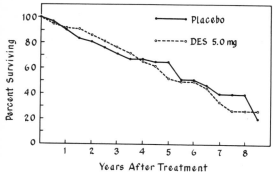

Fig. 2

Survival of stage III prostatic cancer patients. Comparing placebo to diethylstilbestrol 5.0 mg.

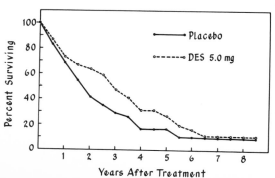

Fig. 3

Survival of stage IV prostatic cancer patients. Comparing placeb to diethylstilbestrol 5.0 mg.

Cause of Death	Placebo	DES 5.0 mg	Total
Carcinoma of the Prostate	28	15	43
Arteriosclerotic Heart Disease (ASHD) with Congestive Heart Failure (CHF)	5	5	10
Myocardial Infarction (MI)	11	16	27
Cerebrovascular Accident (CVA)	4	9	13
Hypertensive Cardiovascular Disease (HCVD)	0	2	2
Pulmonary Embolus	3	3	6
Other	9	9	18
Total Dead/ Total on Study	60/114	59/119	119/233

Fig. 4. Cause of death by primary treatment.

Figure 4 lists the causes of death in both stages combined, along with the primary treatment. The cause of death for each patient was determined by a panel of five investigators. Their decision was based on an independent review of each patient's chart, which contained a copy of the death certificate, the findings at autopsy if such was performed, a summary of the clinical course written by the responsible investigator, a copy of the final hospital summary, or a letter from the attending physician regarding the epicrisis when the patient died at home. The percentage of autopsy in all cases was 42 %.

There was a total of 43 deaths from metastatic carcinoma of the prostate in both Stages III and IV. 28 patients (65 %) received placebo and 15 patients (35 %) received 5.0 mg of stilbestrol daily as their primary treatment. There were 37 deaths from the consequences of arteriosclerotic heart disease. This condition was diagnosed in fatal and non-fatal cases whenever a patient developed angina pectoris, myocardial infarction, or congestive heart failure accompanied by electrocardiographic changes of ischemia. In this group, 16 patients (43 %) were given placebo and 21 men (57 %) received 5.0 mg of stilbestrol daily. Thirteen deaths were due to cerebrovascular accidents. Four of these 13 patients received placebo, and nine were taking 5.0 mg of stilbestrol daily. There were three deaths due to pulmonary embolus in each of the two categories of therapy.

3. Relief of Cancer Symptoms

Before presenting data on the cardiovascular status of prostatic cancer patients before and after therapy, the effects of placebo or 5.0 mg of stilbestrol daily on the prostatic cancer itself should be evaluated. In Stage III patients, clinical improvement was characterized by a 50 % or greater reduction in the size of the prostatic

Primary Treatment	No. of Live Pts.	No. Pts. with ASHD with CHF and/or MI	No. Pts. with CVA	No. Pts. with HCVD with CHF	Percentage of living Pts. with CV Dis.
Placebo	54	5	2	0	13 %
DES 5.0 mg	60	13	1	0	23 %
Total	114	18	3	0	

Fig. 5. Incidence of non-fatal post-treatment cardiovascular disease by primary treatment (includes living patients only).

lesion over the pretreatment status. Stage III prostatic carcinoma did not seem to cause disability other than obstructive symptoms. In addition to a decrease in the extent of prostatic induration, improvement in Stage IV patients was characterized by a decrease in or elimination of bone pain, an increase in strength and appetite, a decrease in prostatic serum acid phosphatase, or a decrease in the density of osseous metastases. The clinical condition was considered worse if there was a 50 % or greater increase in the size of the prostatic lesion, a 50 % or greater increase in prostatic serum acid phosphatase or a change from normal to abnormal [7], an increase in the extent or number of osseous metastases, an increase in bone pain, the appearance of metastases to the soft tissues, or central nervous system involvement, or the development of ureteral obstruction.

In both Stage III and Stage IV, 5.0 mg of stilbestrol daily produced clinical improvement or halted progression of the carcinoma in a higher percentage of men than did placebo. As of May 31, 1969, 36 of 72 Stage III patients (50 %) receiving placebo and 45 of 76 patients (59 %) receiving 5.0 mg of stilbestrol daily were either improved or unchanged. The remaining patients in each treatment group were either worse or dead. Seven of 42 men in Stage IV (17 %) receiving placebo and 12 of 43 men (28 %) receiving 5.0 mg of stilbestrol were either improved or unchanged. The remaining patients in each treatment group were either worse or dead.

4. Cardiovascular status

Figure 5 shows the incidence of non-fatal, post-treatment cardiovascular disease according to primary therapy. Any living patient who had no pretreatment evidence of cardiovascular disease but who developed it following treatment, or who had pretreatment evidence of heart or vascular disease but became worse after going on study, is included in this figure. 7 of 54 living patients (13 %) who were given placebo developed non-fatal cardiovascular disease as opposed to 14 of 60 men (23 %) who

Primary Treatment	No. Pts.	No. Pts. with ASHD with CHF and/or MI	No. Pts. with CVA	No. Pts. with HCVD with CHF	Percentage of Pts. with C–V Disease
Placebo	114	21	6	0	24 %
DES 5.0 mg	119	34	10	2	39 %
Total	233	55	16	2	

Fig. 6. Combined incidence of fatal and non-fatal post-treatment cardiovascular disease by primary treatment.

0   No history of cardiovascular disease; normal ECG.
1   History of cardiovascular disease; not incapacitated; normal ECG.
2   Either no history or history of cardiovascular disease; not incapacitated; abnormal ECG.
3   Definite history of cardiovascular disease; mildly to moderately incapacitated; abnormal ECG.
4   Definite history of cardiovascular disease; severely incapacitated; abnormal ECG.
5   Death due to cardiovascular disease.

Fig. 7. Method of rating clinical cardiovascular status of study patients.

were placed on 5.0 mg of stilbestrol daily. There was no difference between these two groups. When the combined incidence of fatal and non-fatal post-treatment cardiovascular disease is reviewed according to primary treatment, (Figure 6), the difference between the group receiving placebo and that placed on 5.0 mg of stilbestrol becomes apparent ($p < 0.025$). 27 of 114 patients on placebo (24 %) and 46 of 119 men on 5.0 mg of stilbestrol (39 %) developed either fatal or severe, non-fatal cardiovascular disease following treatment.

One may question whether this difference between patients treated with placebo and those treated with estrogen is due to faulty randomization. A method of rating the clinical cardiovascular status of study patients before and after initiation of drug therapy is shown in Figure 7. Rating was done without knowledge of the identity of the study drug, and ranged from 0 (no history of cardiovascular disease, and a normal electrocardiogram) to 5 (death due to cardiovascular disease). After going on the study drug, any period of incapacitation prior to his last examination would cause the patient to receive a 3 or 4 rating. For example, a patient with no previous history of heart disease and a normal pre-treatment electrocardiogram had a severe myocardial infarction one year after going on study. Although the patient might not be severely incapacitated at the year-and-a-half examination, he was severely disabled at the time of the one-year examination and would therefore be assigned a post-treatment rating of 4.

Pre-Treatment

	Placebo			DES 5.0 mg.	
Rating	No. Pts.	Percentage of Total	Rating	No. Pts.	Percentage of Total
0	23	26 %	0	35	37 %
1	10	11 %	1	8	8 %
2	36	41 %	2	31	33 %
3	14	16 %	3	14	15 %
4	5	6 %	4	7	7 %
5	0	0 %	5	0	0 %
Total	88	100 %	Total	95	100 %

Post-Treatment

	Placebo			DES 5.0 mg.	
Rating	No. Pts.	Percentage of Total	Rating	No. Pts.	Percentage of Total
0	15	17 %	0	15	16 %
1	7	8 %	1	8	8 %
2	29	33 %	2	19	20 %
3	15	17 %	3	18	19 %
4	6	7 %	4	9	10 %
5	16	18 %	5	26	27 %
Total	88	100 %	Total	95	100 %

Fig. 8. Rating of clinical cardiovascular status by primary treatment.

Adequate information pertaining to the pre-treatment and post-treatment cardio-vascular status was available on 183 patients. This included 88 men who received placebo and 95 who received 5.0 mg of stilbestrol daily. Information relating to the clinical cardiovascular status of the remaining 50 patients was not available. The distribution of patients according to their primary treatment and clinical cardio-vascular status before and after treatment is shown in Figure 8. There appears to be a fairly even distribution between the two treatment groups except for a higher percentage of estrogen-treated patients with a pre-treatment rating of 0. In the group on placebo, 22 % of the patients were incapacitated before going on study, and 42 % were either incapacitated or dead of cardiovascular disease at some time following treatment. The figures for the group on 5.0 mg of stilbestrol were 22 % incapacitated prior to going on study and 56 % incapacitated or dead of cardiovascular disease at some time following therapy.

0   Normal ECG
1   Benign Abnormalities (bradycardia, infrequent PAC's and PVC's and low voltage
2   Rhythm Disturbances (wandering pacemaker, auricular flutter and fibrillation, paroxysmal
    tachycardia, frequent PVC's and T-wave changes only
3   Blocks (various degrees of AV block, LBBB, RBBB & intraventricular conduction defects
4   Heart Strain (ST-T wave abnormalities, digitalis effect, left axis deviation, left ventricular
    enlargement and strain, right axis deviation, right ventricular enlargement and strain)
5   Old Myocardial Infarction
6   Recent Myocardial Infarction

Fig. 9. Method of rating electrocardiographic changes in study patients [8].

Pre-Treatment

	Placebo			DES 5.0 mg.	
Rating	No. Pts.	Percentage of Total	Rating	No. Pts.	Percentage of Total
0–1	27	34 %	0–1	40	50 %
2	14	18 %	2	6	7 %
3	3	4 %	3	5	6 %
4	26	33 %	4	21	26 %
5	9	11 %	5	9	11 %
6	0	0 %	6	0	0 %
Total	79	100 %	Total	81	100 %

Post-Treatment

	Placebo			DES 5.0 mg.	
Rating	No. Pts.	Percentage of Total	Rating	No. Pts.	Percentage of Total
0–1	21	27 %	0–1	27	33 %
2	6	7 %	2	0	0 %
3	5	6 %	3	5	6 %
4	35	44 %	4	33	41 %
5	10	13 %	5	12	15 %
6	2	3 %	6	4	5 %
Total	79	100 %	Total	81	100 %

Fig. 10. Rating of electrocardiogram by primary treatment.

Electrocardiograms were rated both before and after treatment according to the scale shown in Figure 9 [8]. Rating was from 0 (normal ECG) to 6 (recent myocardial infarction). The immediate pre-treatment electrocardiogram and the worst post-treatment electrocardiogram were rated and recorded. 160 of the 233 patients had both a pre-treatment electrocardiogram and one or more electrocardiograms following treatment. This included 79 men in the group on placebo and 81 in the group receiving 5.0 mg of stilbestrol daily. The distribution of patients according to their primary treatment and pre-treatment and post-treatment electrocardiographic ratings is shown in Figure 10. Again distribution between the two treatment groups appears fairly even except for a higher percentage of estrogen-treated men with a normal pre-treatment tracing. In the group on placebo, 44 % of the patients had a pre-treatment electrocardiographic rating of 4, 5, or 6; after treatment, 60 % of the patients had the same high rating. The figures for the group taking 5.0 mg of stilbestrol daily were 37 % and 61 % respectively.

In studying the group of 183 patients on whom there was adequate pre-treatment and post-treatment information concerning their cardiovascular status, it was noted that 148 men had no pre-treatment history of cardiac or vascular problems. This included 69 patients receiving placebo and 79 receiving 5.0 mg of stilbestrol daily. 27 of 69 patients on placebo, and 14 of 40 estrogen-treated patients, who had normal electrocardiograms before treatment developed an abnormal post-treatment tracing. 28 of 69 men on placebo and 31 of 79 estrogen-treated patients with no previous history of cardiovascular disease showed an abnormal pre-treatment electrocardiogram (usually an ECG rating of 2, 3, or 4) but had no symptoms related to these changes. 22 of the total number of 148 men had no pre-treatment electrocardiogram.

When cardiovascular complications occurred in this group of supposedly healthy men, they were noted on an average of 28 months after the men began to take 5.0 mg of stilbestrol daily, and 50 months after men started on placebo. Figure 11 shows the incidence of fatal and non-fatal cardiovascular complications following treatment according to the status of the pre-treatment electrocardiogram in patients with no previous history of cardiac or vascular problems. When patients with a normal pre-treatment electrocardiogram were given 5.0 mg of stilbestrol daily, they did not develop a higher incidence of cardiovascular complications than did those patients on placebo. When patients with an abnormal pre-treatment electrocardiogram but no previous history of heart disease were treated with 5.0 mg of stilbestrol daily, they were subject to a much higher incidence of cardiovascular complications than were those patients on placebo ($p < 0.005$).

11 of the total number of 233 patients in the study had a post-treatment pulmonary embolus. The embolus was fatal in 6 of 11 patients. Three of 114 patients on placebo (3 %) and 8 of 118 patients on 5.0 mg stilbestrol (7 %) had pulmonary embolism

		According to Pre-Treatment ECG			
Primary Treatment	No. Pts.	No. Pts. with ASHD with CHF and/or MI	No. Pts. with CVA	No. Pts. with Comb. of ASHD & CVA	Percentage of Pt. with C–V Disease
Normal Pre-Treatment ECG					
Placebo	27	4	2	0	22 %
DES 5.0 mg.	40	10	2	1	33 %
Abnormal Pre-Treatment ECG					
Placebo	28	1	0	0	4 %
DES 5.0 mg.	31	10	2	1	42 %
No Pre-Treatment ECG					
Placebo	14	2	0	0	14 %
DES 5.0 mg.	8	2	0	1	38 %

Fig. 11. Incidence of post-treatment cardiovascular disease in living and dead patients with no pre-treatment history of heart disease.

following treatment. All 3 of the patients receiving placebo and 7 of the 8 patients receiving estrogen were hospitalized for pulmonary embolism within the first year following initiation of the study drug.

During the past two years, each patient's blood pressure, pulse, circulation time, electrocardiogram, cardiothoracic ratio, and the presence or absence of peripheral edema were observed and recorded before treatment and at each six-month examination thereafter. It is still too early to assess the changes in these recordings as related to primary treatment and the subsequent development of cardiovascular and cerebrovascular complications.

5. Discussion

When compared to patients receiving placebo, those patients taking 5.0 mg of stilbestrol daily showed an increase in cardiovascular complications and deaths. The 5.0 mg dose of diethylstilbestrol daily did not improve overall survival when compared to placebo in either Stage III or Stage IV patients.

Our study indicates that when 5.0 mg of diethylstilbestrol is given daily to patients with a normal pre-treatment electrocardiogram and no previous history of cardiac disease, the incidence of cardiovascular complications does not differ from that in the group on placebo. However, the 5.0 mg dose of stilbestrol should be administered with caution to patients having an abnormal pre-treatment electrocardiogram, even though they give no past history of cardiovascular problems. A large number of supposedly "healthy" men had pre-treatment electrocardiographic changes such as left bundle branch block, left ventricular hypertrophy, and non-specific ST-T wave changes, and it was this group that so often developed cardiovascular problems when given estrogen. We must decide whether the increased risk of cardiovascular and cerebrovascular problems associated with the 5.0 mg dose is compensated for by the beneficial effects of the estrogen on the carcinoma.

When estrogen becomes necessary for the treatment of symptomatic carcinoma of the prostate, what is the optimum dose? In the original reports of *Herbst* [9] and *Huggins* [10], patients with metastatic cancer responded to a 1.0 mg dose of diethylstilbestrol. Patients in both Stage III and Stage IV in our second study have responded favorably to 1.0 mg dosage. Apparently this smaller dose is oncologically active. Our early studies indicate that it does not contribute to the development of cardiovascular and cerebrovascular complications as much as the 5.0 mg dosage does.

Doe and others [12, 14] have reported the effects of estrogen on certain serum proteins. Corticosteroid-binding globulin, 17-hydroxycorticosteroids, ceruloplasmin, beta-glucouronidase, and plasminogen predictably rise when small doses of estrogen are administered, and this rise in post-treatment values is related to the dose. Plasminogen activation ordinarily declines in the aging male. Estrogen has been reported to suppress plasminogen activity. Conversion of plasminogen to plasmin is probably essential in preventing fibrin deposition on the endothelial lining of blood vessels. *Doe* and his associates have found that plasminogen rises more in estrogen-treated patients than in men receiving placebo. This rise in plasminogen is roughly related to the size of the dose and may reflect decreased activation of plasminogen. Cholesterol values have been unpredictable in their response to administration of estrogen, in this study. None of these changes in serum proteins or lipids has been of value, as yet, in predicting which patients were destined to develop heart disease or strokes.

References

[1] Veterans Administration Cooperative Urological Research Group: Treatment and survival of patients with cancer of the prostate. Surg. Gynec. & Obst., 124, 1011–1017, 1967.

[2] Veterans Administration Cooperative Urological Research Group: Carcinoma of the prostate: treatment comparisons. J. Urol., 98, 516–522, 1967.

[3] *Hanash, K. A., Taylor, W. F., Greene, L. F., Kottke, B. A.* and *Titus, J. L.*: Estrogen therapy for carcinoma of the prostate and atherosclerotic cardiovascular disease: a clinical-pathologic study. Presented at the Annual Meeting of the American Urological-Association, San Francisco, California, May 11–15, 1969.

76   G. T. Mellinger and C. Blackard

[4] *Kalman, S. M.:* Effects of oral contraceptives. Ann. Rev. Pharmacol., **9**, 363–378, 1969.

[5] Medical Research Council Subcommittee: Risk of thromboembolic disease in women taking oral contraceptives. Brit. M. J., **2**, 355–359, 1967.

[6] *Cutler, S. J.:* Computation of survival rates. Nat. Cancer Inst. Monogr., **15**, 381–385, 1964.

[7] Veterans Administration Cooperative Urological Research Group: Factors in the prognosis of carcinoma of the prostate; a cooperative study. J. Urol., **100**, 59–65, 1968.

[8] *Bailar, J. C.,* III: National Cancer Institute. Personal communication.

[9] *Herbst, W. P.:* The effects of estradiol dipropionate and diethyl stilbestrol on malignant prostatic tissue. Tr. Am. A. Genito-Urin. Surgeons, **34**, 195–202, 1941.

[10] *Huggins, C.* and *Hodges, C. V.:* Studies on prostatic cancer: I. The effect of castration, of estrogen and of androgen injection on serum phosphatases in metastatic carcinoma of the prostate. Cancer Res., **1**, 293–297, 1941.

[11] Veterans Administration Cooperative Urological Research Group: Estrogen treatment for cancer of the prostate: early results with three doses of diethylstilbestrol and placebo. Submitted for publication.

[12] *Musa, B. U., Seal, U. S.* and *Doe, R. P.:* Elevation of certain plasma proteins in man following estrogen administration: a dose-response relationship. J. Clin. Endocrinol., **25**, 1163–1166, 1965.

[13] *Doe, R. P., Mellinger, G. T., Swaim, W. F.* and *Seal, U. S.:* Estrogen dosage effects on serum proteins: a longitudinal study. J. Clin. Endocrinol., **27**, 1081–1086, 1967.

[14] *Musa, B. U., Doe, R. P.* and *Seal, U. S.:* Serum protein alterations produced in women by synthetic estrogens. J. Clin. Endocrinol., **27**, 1463–1469, 1967.

Discussion

A.-A. Kollwitz: I want to congratulate Dr. *Mellinger* on his very good results with a 55 % 5 year survival for all kinds of treatment. As Prof. *Brosig* just pointed out, our results, and those in the older American literature are much worse. May I give you the results of 311 patients with prostatic cancer in our department. 2/3 of patients were without metastases and 1/3 had metastases. 28 patients of these 311 underwent radical prostatectomy. 144 were treated by orchiectomy and oestrogen, 116 by oestrogens alone, and the rest underwent orchiectomy only, or was untreated.

The average age of our patients was 72. With radical prostatectomies we had a 5 year survival of 60 %; with orchiectomy and oestrogens a survival of 40 %; with oestrogens alone of 27 %; and untreated patients survived in only 11 % of the cases. You see that orchiectomy and oestrogens in our experience, as well as in the older American literature and in the German statistics by *Gaca* and *Röhl* are much better than oestrogens alone.

The 5 year survival of patients with metastases, treated by orchiectomy and oestrogens was 20 %; with oestrogens alone it was 7 %.

W. E. Goodwin: In the United States one of the important things has been discussion of the Veterans' Administration study. There have been some critical remarks made about it. I would like to ask Prof. *Scott* to make a brief critique for us on the Veterans' study.

W. W. Scott: I am not sure I can fill that bill, but I will try. I enjoyed Dr. *Mellinger's* summary very much and I am more pleased with it than when I read the first report in May 1967. I am still concerned about the higher than 30 % exclusion before treatment, and the fact that evaluation was based on initial treatment only, although the treatment was frequently changed. Also, the number of patients at risk in any one year is not given. His retrospective studies, at the Minneapolis Veteran's Hospital, concerning the cardiovascular studies *before* treatment, which I did not see in the first report, seems to me to have been made *after* treatment, or during the retrospective study, and hence, are not objective. Finally, there have been good double blind studies in the United States which indicate that a second coronary occlusion is *less* likely if the patient is on oestrogen compared to placebo. I will be glad to furnish you with these data. Finally, in the patient's point system, I wanted to know if one is assigned fewer or more points for going to church. All these points, I think, indicate the need for more knowledge about the biological potential of these tumors, before we can evaluate *any* of these treatments.

W. E. Goodwin: There is one more person who has asked to discuss Dr. *Mellinger's* paper, before we ask Dr. *Mellinger* for a rebuttle, and that is Prof. *Balogh* from Hungary.

F. Balogh: I should like to ask Prof. *Mellinger:* Isn't 5 mg of oestrogen per day too little? We give 20 mg oestrogen per day, for 6 weeks. How can the placebo be dangerous for the patient, because it should have no action upon the patient. The placebo has no therapeutic effect.

Now I should like to give our results. Our attitude can be summarised as follows. If, in an operative specimen of a prostatic adenoma, there is an incidental finding of a malignant focus at the histological examination, no subsequent operation should be performed, but oestrogen administration should be started since there may be some response to hormones. Follow-up examinations should be instituted at 6 week intervals and if there is any progress in the condition an orchiectomy should be performed and oestrogen therapy continued. If occult prostatic cancer is discovered during the course of the transurethral resection, oestrogen therapy is commenced and a radical transvesical prostatectomy performed. During the last 15 years in two clinics at Budapest and Pecs, 46 patients have been treated in our institute according to the above principle. 30 of these patients have replied to a questionnaire, 28 of them, 63 %, have survived for more than 5 years. 23 of these are symptom free. In 5 cases there is difficulty in micturition and there are symptoms suggesting recurrence. The survival time is not worse than the survival time of patients in the same age group, but without cancer. We feel therefore that no radical operation is necessary for occult prostatic cancer which can be regarded as a local process and *not* especially malignant.

G. Jönsson: Dr. *Mellinger,* I have a question, In your conclusions you said that we should not give oestrogen to patients before they have severe symptoms. When you say oestrogen, you mean stilboestrol, which is the form used in your investigations. Do you have the same opinion about the conjugated, natural oestrogens, regarding side effects? I think that is a very important question.

Another question. You must have seen many patients with severe pain, and with extensive metastases in stage IV. Have the pain and metastases ever disappeared with a placebo?

A. Sigel: Dr. *Mellinger,* whether your results with placebo or DDS (Diethyl-stilboestrol-diphosphate) are right or wrong, when you started your investigations, you could not predict your results for several years. Your results could have been the contrary. What was your ethical standpoint?

F. Schroeder: I would like to refer to one group of Dr. *Belt's* data which came out of the IBM machine and which, I think, may be significant. There were 254 patients who were dead at the time that the study was done. Of these 254, 92 for some reason or other did not receive the usual dose of oestrogen that Dr. *Belt* gives. Thus a total of 37.4% received no oestrogen. In this group of 254 patients, 97 patients died from cerebrovascular incidents – strokes. Of these 97,28 patients, or 38.2 %, did not receive oestrogen. Interestingly enough, the figures of 38.2 % and 37.4 % are almost identical. This does not reflect the fact that the patient had or did not have oestrogen, *but* the distribution of patients in the groups, with oestrogens and without. So it cannot be said that this large number of patients who died from CVAS died because they had oestrogens.

G. T. Mellinger: Question one: " How do I explain our good survival rate compared to the previous studies? "

Well, in the last 10 years antibiotics and many other treatments have been developed which were not available before. In some of the previous studies patients died from infections, or they may have died from coronaries. Not as many people die *now* from heart disease, as died previously. The incidence may be as high, but our treatments are better. Our results are, actually, over 6 years. 40 % of stage II patients are still alive at the end of 6 years. Now we have a number of them still alive after 10 years, but this number is small of course. Strangely enough, over 20 % of stage IV patients who have an elevated acid phosphatase, or definite osseous metastases are still alive at the end of 6 years. Surprisingly, quite a few of them are alive at the end of 10 years. I think this is due to antibiotics and other treatments which have improved.

The second question concerns the supposed effect of oestrogens (I say *supposed*) in diminishing the number of heart attacks. Dr. *Scott,* I have read many of these studies, but there are faults in each. For example, Dr. *Marmeston's* study, only considered a coronary significant if it occurred 6 months after oestrogen began. She maintained that any coronary occurring during the first 6 months could not be prevented and that it took *too* long for the oestrogen to affect it. Each of these studies has a fault. We're hoping that our studies will reveal this.

Question three is: "Why do we have rejects?" We could eliminate rejects by including anyone in our study who has had previous treatment. I do not think any study in which we have patients who have been treated before could be significant. This accounts for the vast majority of our rejects. There are also some who turned down treatment. This raises the question – what happens to these patients? The patients who turn down treatment, are they sicker or better patients? Well, we also followed them up. By the way, let me tell you about our follow-up. Each patient is seen every 6 months. He is seen 3 months and 6 months after beginning treatment, and every 6 months thereafter, as long as he is able to travel or to be seen. At each visit blood is drawn to estimate haemoglobin, and serum acid phosphatase. He then has an intravenous pyelogram. He has a complete bone survey. Then he is examined by the examiner, who examines his prostate. At the same time certain other chemical studies are performed, depending on which of the studies it is, whether to estimate cholesterol, BUN's, the various proteins, caeruloplasmin or plasma cortisols. There are about 14 different chemical tests.

As for our "drop-off" percentage. It works as I said. – We have a certain percentage who do change their treatment. They change, for several reasons, the first one being, of course, that they are sick. A certain percentage of them are seen elsewhere, and their doctor does not like their treatment. He says, "I think all of my patients should receive treatment thus and thus."

Something was mentioned about the difference using different oestrogens. Would there be a different effect? We pose ourselves the same question. Therefore we have started a new study, which began on 1st June. It is Prostate III. In this study, we will be treating stage I and II exactly as we are in this study. This is, as you may say, a continuation of the study for stages I and II. Stages III and IV are receiving one of four treatments. The first treatment is stilboestrol, I mg daily. This is a control. The second treatment is progesterone, 3 mg a day. The fourth treatment is Premarin, 2.5 mg a day. I don't think Premarin makes much difference. I don't think Premarin will be the drug, but we don't know this, so we have to find out. That is the only way we will find out. I do believe that use of oestradiol is promising. Now this is not in any control. Thus is a group of patients whom I have treated on my own, and not concerned with the study at all. I have some patients on whom I have used oestroduran, which as you know is an injectable preparation of oestradiol. Oestradiol apparently does not affect the serum proteins at all. It produces maximal breast changes, and it apparently affects the prostate very well. I would have liked to have put it on this Prostate III study, however it must be injected, and this prohibits its use in quite a lot of the patients. It is very difficult to call patients in from 1500 miles away to inject them once a month. So we have not introduced this in the study.

Is 5 mg too small a dose? I used to think before this study began, that 15 mg was an ideal dose, Now I think 5 mg is too large a dose. I think we have shown fairly well that 1 mg is probably the best dose. Many people have said this before; but there has been no unanimity on this. If you are going to use stilboestrol, 1 mg is the best dose.

As for placebo — the reason we use placebo is as a control. I don't think the study would have meant anything, if we had not used a placebo. It was difficult to use a placebo. We did not expect these results. It was very difficult. It caused great ethical problems. We considered this, for 9 months, before we finally decided, this was the only way. If we wanted to find anything out we had to use a placebo. I am very glad we did. It was much easier in Prostate II to use it, because then I began to believe that maybe radical prostatectomy was not the best treatment for stage I.

As for biopsy, I did not say it, because I think it goes without saying — all of our patients had biopsies prior to treatment. Several of them have also had biopsies after treatment. Our experience with repeated biopsies is that on patients who have had an orchiectomy, there is not very much effect upon the histology of the prostate (although with oestrogens there are very marked effects).

H. Marberger: Dr. *Jönsson* asked you what you would do if the patient is in pain. Do you switch to other drugs?

G. T. Mellinger: In stage IV? This is the main reason why we have taken patients off our studies, because of persistence of pain. Ethically we can not let a man suffer. However, some patients did improve on placebo and the placebo is, in this case, lactose and it was used as a control.

N. Brock: Whenever you feel that the cardiovascular side-effects of stilboestrol are caused by the oestrogen or hormonal activity of such compounds, it seems to be advisable to try a compound as e. g. stilboestrol diphosphate with a much lower hormonal activity. No doubt that it is more complicated to use a drug which has to be injected i. v., but since there is a chance that this drug will not produce the above mentioned side-effects, I feel that a comparative study between conventional oestrogens and stilboestrol diphosphate should be conducted.

G. T. Mellinger: We have not used it as a part of this study at all. However, on certain other patients I have used it. I have not seen any effects that are not comparable to stilboestrol. When stilboestrol no longer has an effect, I no longer get effects from the stilboestrol diphosphate.

J. Frick: We checked two compounds – ethinyl oestradiol and megoestrol acetate – as to testosterone supression in the plasma. We checked this by measuring the plasma testosterone.

We implanted silastic capsules. These implants had a length of 20 mm. and the hole had a diameter of 0.84 mm. These implants were filled with 20 mg of ethinyl oestradiol, or 30 mg of megoestrol acetate. The releasing factor per 24 hours from this implant was 20 μg for ethinyl oestradiol and 30 μg for megoestrol acetate. The basic research on these implants was done by Dr. *Segal* and Dr. *Kincl* at the Population Council of the Rockefeller University.

We implanted these capsules subcutaneously.

After the implantation of two silastic capsules containing ethinyl oestradiol, together about 40 mg, we saw a fall in the plasma testosterone. After 10 days in both patients we got a decrease of the plasma testosterone to a remarkable degree.

From three more patients in whom we implanted two silastic capsules, only one patient showed no sign of decrease. The other two patients showed a marked decrease.

Then we tried megoestrol acetate. It is a progesteronelike substance. When we implanted these capsules with megoestrol acetate (here we implanted 60 mg) we could see no effect after 10 days.

We checked two more patients, with 120 mg of megoestrol acetate and saw no effect.

Three more patients were implanted with 180 mg of megoestrol acetate and we could see no effect after 10 days. The plasma testosterone level did not decrease.

Seven patients with carcinoma of the prostate received different kinds of treatment. Only two patients – the first one with 0.03 and the last one with 0.02 – had practically no testosterone in the blood. The levels in patients No. 3 and 4 were low. Perhaps testosterone is produced by the adrenals, but No. 5, 2 and 6 had (after orchiectomy and regular treatment with oestrogen) too high a level of plasma testosterone. We have no explanation for this fact; perhaps the prostatic tissue can convert steroids to testosterone. I think Dr. *Walsh* can give us another theory for this occurrence. I would ask Dr. *Walsh* to comment on these points.

P. Walsh: We have been interested in the effect of oestrogens on the control of gonadotropins in the male. We have investigated the effect of oral ethinyl oestradiol on the suppression of radioimmunoassable LH in the serum of castrated male patients. We found clearly that 40–50 μg per day of ethinyl oestradiol was the lowest dose of oestrogen which suppressed LH to the normal range. So it appears that this is the lowest dose of oestrogen, at least from these two studies, which effects the lowering of circulating androgens in the male. With respect to the patients of yours with elevated plasma testosterone levels following castration, the studies of *Young* and *Kent* demonstrated immeasurable levels of testosterone in most castrated patients up to 5 years post castration. Your patients, as I understand, had subcapsular orchiectomy, and I wonder whether there is sufficient Leydig function to account for this increase in plasma testosterone. This is an alternative explanation, as opposed to androgen production by the prostate.

Methods of Hormonal Treatment including Orchiectomy and Adrenalectomy

W. W. Scott

Hopkins Hospital, Baltimore, Maryland, USA

Summary: Hormonal therapy was introduced in 1941 based on laboratory data which suggested that prostatic cancer might atrophy if androgen production is diminished by castration or inhibited by estrogen administration. It soon became evident that there must be an extra gonadal source of androgen — the adrenals. Adrenalectomy, however, was impractical until cortisone became available in 1951.

Since that time, only few reports have been published so that it is difficult till now to assess the value of adrenalectomy for prostatic cancer.

Results are given of the author's own analyses on steroid response related to hormonal therapy of prostatic cancer.

Furthermore a report is added concerning a method of establishing portal drainage of left adrenal blood, and removing the right adrenal.

As indicated in your program, I have been invited to open the discussion on methods of hormonal treatment, including orchiectomy and adrenalectomy. In endeavoring to prepare this introduction, I also noted that Dr. *C. V. Hodges* was scheduled to talk on the basis of hormonal treatment, Dr. *George T. Mellinger* to cover the results of hormonal treatment and Mr. *J. D. Fergusson* to review the results of hypophysectomy. Also, I noted that the Saturday morning session is to be devoted to a subject dear to me, *Experiences with Cyproterone acetate and Related Substances in the Treatment of Disease of the Prostate.*

It seemed to me, therefore, that I could best serve by taking up where Dr. *Hodges* left off, tracing the rationale for adrenalectomy and perhaps presenting the results which admittedly are scanty.

As Dr. *Hodges* has said, the rationale for hormonal therapy was based on laboratory data which suggested that prostatic cancer epithelium is an "overgrowth" of normal, adult prostatic epithelium and might atrophy — as does normal, adult prostatic epithelium — if androgen production is diminished by castration or inhibited by estrogen administration.

Shortly after the introduction of hormonal therapy in 1941, it became evident that some patients — perhaps one-third — failed to show any response to castration

Manuscript received: 5 December 1969

Case No.	Subject	Age	Preoperative Average of 17-Ketosteroid, mg. per day	Lowest Post-Operative level of 17-Ketosteroid, mg. per day	Time Since Castration, days	Highest Postoperative Level of 17-Ketosteroid, mg. per day	Time Since Castration, days	Last Value of 17-Ketosteroid Observed, mg. per day	Total No. of Post-Operative Days Observed	Total No. of Urine Samples Extracted
1	G.N.A.	53	3.6	0.4	3	15.9	12	9.4	49	8
2	A.E.D.	58	5.7	3.8	14	9.8	233	9.8	233	16
3	J.D.J.	58	7.3	5.0	10	10.4	187	10.4	187	15
4	F.M.	47	10.8	5.3	3	15.4	27	11.1	183	8
5	J.H.Q.	80	5.3	2.1	2	7.3	86	7.3	86	20
6	G.T.R.	56	10.8	7.4	100	19.3	4	14.0	128	15
7	J.T.	67	11.7	3.1	13	12.3	67	12.3	67	18
8	J.J.T.	70	4.2	2.0	3	10.2	115	7.8	183	10
9	W.W.	67	7.0	1.6	3	31.4	175	24.4	200	20
10	J.A.Y.	71	9.8	4.2	7	7.5	106	7.5	106	10
Average		63	7.62	3.49	15.8 (6.5)[1]	13.95	101.2	11.4	142.2	14

[1] Average time since castration excluding G.T.R.

Fig. 1. 17-ketosteroid excretion in the urine of patients with prostatic cancer before and after castration [1].

or estrogen therapy, and that in the remaining two-thirds, relapse was almost inevitable. This suggested to us that if the original basis for hormonal therapy was correct that there must be an extra gonadal source of androgen — most likely the adrenals.

In 1942, Dr. *Cornelius Vermeulen* and I reported our studies on urinary 17-ketosteroid excretion in patients with prostatic cancer before and after castration [1]. It must be recalled that in those early days we measured only *total* urinary 17-ketosteroids, and serum testosterone could not be measured. Qualitative studies of urinary 17-ketosteroids were made later and will be discussed briefly shortly.

Figure 1 reproduces Figure 4 of this Study. Before castration, the levels of total urinary 17-ketosteroids in these 10 patients averaged 7.6 mg. per 24 hours. After castration, the levels fell in all patients. This fall was not sustained. Levels gradually rose in all but one patient (# 10.-J. A. Y.) to a level higher than before castration.

Figure 2 is Figure 1 from this study and indicates these changes graphically.

Fully aware that the level of total urinary 17-ketosteroids is not an accurate reflection of androgen production, we felt, nevertheless, that the postcastration rise in these steroids did suggest androgen production by the adrenal and that adrenal androgens might be responsible for postcastration relapse.

Such considerations prompted *Charles Huggins* and your speaker to perform bilateral adrenalectomy in the early 1940's. The results in 4 patients were reported in 1945 [2]. At that time it was almost impossible to maintain life after adrenalectomy. Cortisone was not available, and adrenal cortical extracts were impotent. DOCA and salt were the only worthwhile agents of the time. These 4 men survived adrenalectomy for 1.5, 1.5, 11 and 116 days, an insufficient period in all but one to permit us to make any deductions.

Figure 3 represents Figure 4 of this study and shows the values for urinary 17-ketosteroids in the longest survivor. Total and α-ketonic urinary steroids fell promptly after bilateral adrenalectomy to very low levels, and biologic assay showed no androgen in the urine on postoperative day 80. The patient's prostatic cancer progressed.

This early study prompted us to conclude that adrenalectomy — without cortisone — was impractical in the treatment of postcastration relapse. It did suggest that the extra gonadal source of androgens was the adrenal and that certain prostatic cancers were androgen independent.

Adrenalectomy for inoperable prostatic cancer was revived in 1951 by *Huggins* and *Bergenstal* [3]. By then cortisone was available, and it became possible to maintain life in the adrenalectomized man.

In 1954, *Hudson* and I [4] reviewed all reports in the literature of adrenalectomy for prostatic cancer. Time does not permit presentation of these data. However, as an example of what can be expected let us refer to a representative group of 10

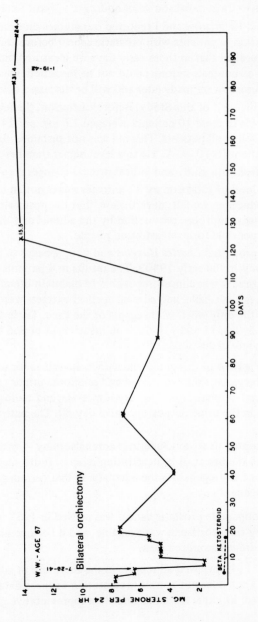

Fig. 2. Postcastration fall and subsequent rise of urinary 17-ketosteroids in patients with disseminated prostatic cancer [1].

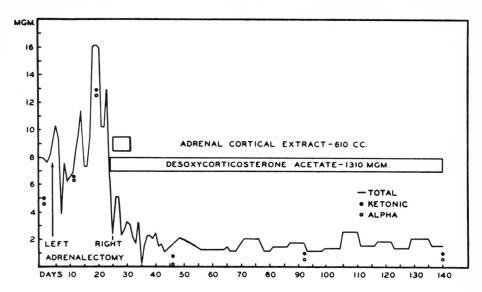

Fig. 3. Decrease of alpha, ketonic and total urinary 17-ketosteroids following complete adrenalectomy with survival for 116 days [2].

patients adrenalectomized for prostatic cancer and reported on in 1952 by *West, Hollander, Whitmore, Randall* and *Pearson* of the Memorial Hospital in New York City [5]. "Three died in the immediate postoperative period, one from cerebral hemorrhage (2 days), one from carcinomatosis (11 days) and one from myocardial infarction (21 days). Six of the remaining seven died within 33 to 294 days after adrenalectomy, two from adrenal insufficiency and four from cancer." The remaining patient was living at the writing of this addendum, his 159th postoperative day. Quoting further: "All seven patients had temporary subjective improvement varying from 14 to 210 days, averaging 82 days. Only two of the seven had objective improvement lasting 90 and 133 days. The most striking beneficial response to adrenalectomy was relief of pain." There has not been a publication from the Huggins laboratory on adrenalectomy for prostatic cancer since that of *Huggins* and *Bergenstal* [6], to be found in Cancer Research for 1952, and the results in this series of seven patients are quite comparable to those of the Memorial Hospital group.

Our results and those of others have been quite similar, and a recent review of the literature revealed very few reports of adrenalectomy for prostatic cancer. This is in sharp contrast to the many cases reported of adrenalectomy for disseminated breast cancer in women.

We believe that at present there are insufficient data to permit one to assess the value of adrenalectomy in the treatment of disseminated prostatic cancer. The somewhat favorable response of female breast cancer to adrenalectomy perhaps suggests that more extensive trials are indicated in prostatic cancer.

While the *Huggins* laboratory was concentrating its efforts on adrenalectomy, we at *Johns Hopkins* were concentrating on hypophysectomy, as a treatment of relapse following castration-estrogen therapy, and were studying steroid response to therapy in prostatic cancer with the newer methods which were developed by *Dobriner* and *Gallagher* [7, 8, 9]. Hypophysectomy will be discussed by Mr. *J. D. Fergusson,* and I shall not review our experiences which were published in 1962 [10]. However, I will review our work on steroid response, because it has a direct bearing on possible mechanisms of action of hormonal therapy of prostatic cancer.

With the development of infrared analysis of extracts of urine, it became possible to both *quantitate* and *qualitate* urinary 17-ketosteroids. In so-doing one can separate "androgen metabolites" from "corticoid metabolites", and evidence suggests that the former are derived from both the gonads and the adrenal and the latter from the adrenal only.

In 1957 we [11] published the results of such analyses in a series of patients with prostatic cancer. In summary:

(1)   "Androgen" metabolites fall after castration;

(2)   "Corticoid" and "androgen" metabolites may rise when a patient relapses after castration;

(3)   The effect of ACTH on both "androgen" and "corticoid" metabolites is markedly enhanced by castration;

(4)   Stilbestrol causes a fall in "androgen" and "corticoid" metabolites in the intact and castrate patient;

(5)   Cortisone can effectively eliminate "androgen" metabolites in the urine;

(6)   In our limited series of patients, the clinical state has invariably paralleled the chemical state.

Figure 4 reproduces Table 6 of our article referred to previously. Here we see a fairly close parallel between the ratio of the biologically active urinary androgen — androsterone — and the biologically inactive epimere — etiocholanolone — and the clinical state of the patient.

Again, we appreciate that androgen excretion does not necessarily measure androgen production, but we contend that it frequently approximates it. Thus, it seems to us

Patient	Ratio: androsterone etiocholanolone	Therapy			Months followed	Present state
		castrate	estrogen	cortisone		
F.P. 56 C.M.	0.87	.X	X	X	17	relapse
R.D. 56 W.M.	0.82	X	X	X	16	dead
A.S. 70 C.M.	0.81	X			10	dead
F.J. 60 C.M.	0.69	X	X		6	relapse
R.C. 55 C.M.	0.54		X		7	well
J.M. 65 C.M.	0.52		X		6	well
J.E. 60 C.M.	0.51	X	X*		15	well
J.R. 61 C.M.	0.38	X	X*		14	well
W.J. 70 C.M.	0.34	X			6	well
E.B. 74 C.M.	0.25		X		7	no relapse

* Given without indication

Fig. 4. Correlation between tendency to relapse and ratio of urinary androsterone: etiocholanolone [11].

that one logical approach to therapy for the patient with prostatic cancer, who has relapsed on castration-estrogen therapy is to search for means of suppressing or eliminating an extragonadal source of androgens.

While working in the Brady Laboratories, Drs. *John Grayhack* and *Page Harris* [12] reported a method for establishing portal drainage of adrenal venous blood in dogs. This is illustrated in Figure 5 (Figure 1 of [12]). The right adrenal was excised at the same time.

A wealth of evidence from our laboratories both before and since has indicated that the liver inactivates androgens, even if severe liver damage is present, but not cortisone. *Grayhack* and *Harris* then proceeded to establish portal drainage of left adrenal blood in five humans with disseminated prostatic cancer, removing the right adrenal. They were successful in four of the five patients, and in none of the four who had a successful shunt, as evidenced by good function of the left kidney on an intravenous pyelogram, was cortisone necessary to maintain life. Figure 6 is the I. V. P. of one of the four. Unfortunately, none of these four with successful shunts showed any great improvement in his clinical course.

This idea still intrigues me and merits further investigation. More recently we [13] have shown that portal diversion of testicular (and adrenal) blood in dogs abolishes prostatic secretion for as long as collateral circulation does not develop. Figure 7 (Figure 3 of [13]) illustrates this effect; i. e., almost total abolition of pilocarpine-stimulated prostatic secretion in a dog with a prostatic fistula after protacaval transposition. This lasted for 200 days, or until collateral circulation developed.

Hopefully, my remarks have served as an introduction to a discussion of adrenalectomy in the treatment of relapse following castration-estrogen therapy. This was

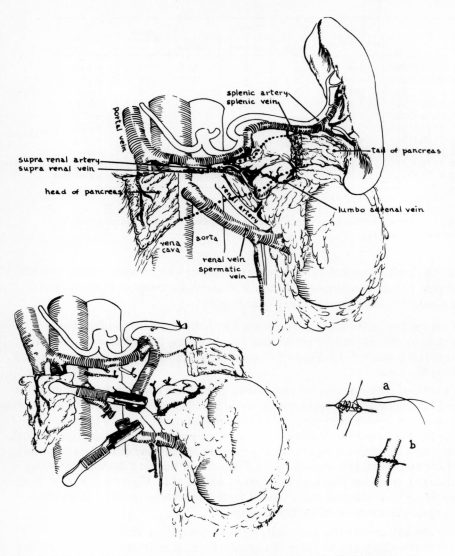

Fig. 5. Schematic drawing of pre- and postoperative views of renal-splenic anastomosis illustrating dependence of adrenal on renal pedicle for its blood supply. Insets a and b show vascular anastomosis [12].

my purpose. Personally, I know of no way of determining effectiveness short of increasing our experience by doing more. As secondary therapies to oophorectomy, both bilateral adrenalectomy and hypophysectomy have proved to be of real value in the treatment of breast cancer, and it is possible that a similar response would be found if more patients with disseminated prostatic cancer in relapse after castration-estrogen therapy were subjected to hypophysectomy or adrenalectomy.

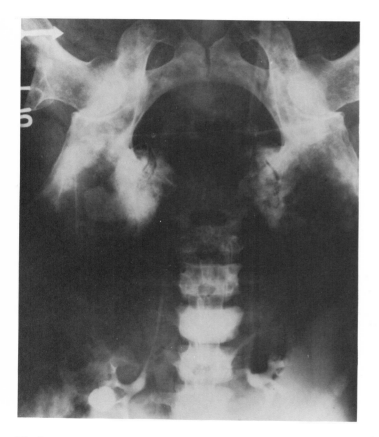

Fig. 6. Intravenous pyelogram of a patient with disseminated prostatic cancer who underwent creation of a vascular shunt which established portal drainage of adrenal venous blood. Note good function of the left kidney indicating a patent shunt. The round density overlying the left kidney is a calcified mesenteric lymph node.

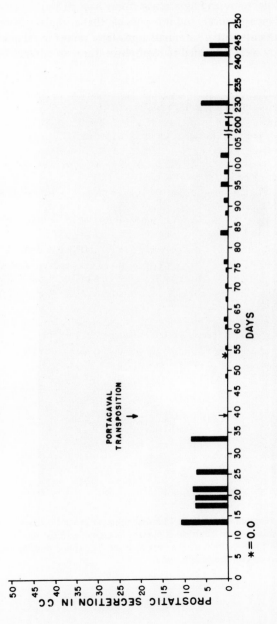

Fig. 7. Reduction and recovery in the volume of prostatic secretion incident to portal diversion of testicular blood and subsequent development of collateral circulation [13].

References

[1] *Scott, W. W.* and *Vermeulen, C.:* Studies on prostatic cancer. V. Excretion of 17-Ketosteroids, estrogens and gonadotropins before and after castration. J. Clin. Endocrinol. **2**, 450–456, 1942.

[2] *Huggins, C.* and *Scott, W. W.:* Bilateral adrenalectomy in prostatic cancer: Clinical features and urinary excretion of 17-ketosteroids and estrogen. Annals Surg. **122**, 1031–1041, 1945.

[3] *Huggins, C.* and *Bergenstal, D. M.:* Surgery of the adrenals. JAMA 147, 101, 1951.

[4] *Scott, W. W.* and *Hudson, P. B.:* Surgery of the adrenal glands. Ed.: *L. R. Dragstedt.* Charles C. Thomas, Publisher, Springfield, Illinois, 1954.

[5] *West, C. D., Hollander, V. P., Whitmore, W. F., Jr., Randall, H. T.* and *Pearson, O. H.:* The effect of bilateral adrenalectomy upon neoplastic disease in man. Cancer **5**, 1009–1018, 1952.

[6] *Huggins, C.* and *Bergenstal, D. M.:* Inhibition of human mammary and prostatic cancers by adrenalectomy. Cancer Resch. **12**, 134–141, 1952.

[7] *Liebermann, S., Mond, B.* and *Smyles, E.:* Recent progress in hormone research **9**, 113–129, 1954.

[8] *Dobriner, K., Kappas, A., Rhoads, C. P.* and *Gallagher, T. F.:* J. Clin. Invest. **32**, 940–949, 1954.

[9] *Lieberman, S.* and *Dobriner, K.:* Recent progress in hormone research 3, 71–101, 1948.

[10] *Scott, W. W.* and *Schirmer, H. K. A.:* "Hypophysectomy for disseminated prostatic cancer" in: On Cancer and Hormones, University of Chicago Press, Chicago, 1962.

[11] *Burt, F. B., Finney, R. P.* and *Scott, W. W.:* Steroid response to therapy in prostatic cancer. J. Urol. 77, 485–491, 1957.

[12] *Grayhack, J. T.* and *Harris, A. P.:* A method for establishing portal drainage of adrenal venous blood in dogs with metabolic studies included. J. Urol. 73, 1–16, 1955.

[13] *Robson, M. C.* and *Scott, W. W.:* Effect of portal diversion of testicular blood on prostatic secretion in the dog. Invest. Urol. 2, 92–98, 1964.

Total Perineal Prostatectomy in 398 Patients with Cancer of the Prostate

E. Belt and F. H. Schröder

University of California, Department of Surgery/Urology, Los Angeles, USA
University of California, Departments of Biology and Urology, San Diego, USA

Summary: A series of 398 total perineal prostatectomies for cancer of the prostate is presented and analyzed. All patients were at least followed for five years, 303 for 10–15 and 218 for over 15 years. This series is different from others because 105 patients over age 70 and 123 patients with tumorextension through the prostatic capsule were included. The rates of survival for the three groups were

5–10	years	71.8 %
10–15	years	38.6 %
over 15	years	21.6 %.

The large number of patients makes it possible to compare survival in five year age-groups to the life expectancy of the American male of the same age. This method is used to study the dependence of survival of our patients with prostatic carcinoma on age, tumor extension and histological grade. Both, age and tumor extension significantly influence the time of survival. In the younger patients the tumor killed 53.8 % or 7 of 13, whereas the overall mortality from recurrent or metastatic carcinoma was only 12.8 % or 53 of 398 patients. The data on grading are presently incomplete and do not allow final conclusions.

Considering all data presented, there is no doubt, that in the cases of prostatic cancer analyzed in this study, life expectancy is markedly decreased in all age-groups in spite of total prostatectomy. This tumor is regardless of age, stage or grade by no means a harmless disease.

In considering our data it should be noted that our selection of patients has been a little broader than in the groups of cases selected for this operation throughout the United States. Our wider selection has been in regard to age. We are including 105 patients of the ages of 70 or over. Our average age is 65.6. We are also including 123 patients in whom local extension beyond the capsule of the prostate was recognized on digital rectal examination of the prostate pre-operatively. Both of these differences would tend statistically to diminish the survival time in this large group of 398 patients.

Detection of tumor extension beyond the capsule of the prostate is tricky at best. Upon rectal examination we recorded our belief that the cancer was confined within the prostate in 245 of the patients subsequently operated upon. Our pathologist

Manuscript received: 14 November 1969

reported that in only 166 of these patients was the cancer actually confined within the capsule. Thus extension in 79 of these patients was found unexpectedly.

In this series, 214 patients underwent perineal exploration and total perineal prostatectomy without prior tissue diagnosis. No diagnostic error was made in this group operated upon without the advantage of prior biopsy.

Broders' classification by the pathologist in grading the tumors we removed is not recorded for all of our patients; however, in those patients in whom careful grading was carried out the grade of the tumor did not seem to have a significant influence on survival.

Regarding the appearance of metastatic disease with the passage of time after prostatectomy: In our series of 398 patients, generalized metastases developed in only 67 patients or 16.8 %. 38 of these 398 patients developed local nodules, some of which were extirpated postoperatively. In these no further metastases occurred. However, 53 of the 67 patients who developed recognized metastases are dead. 14 are still living. 13 of the 38 patients with local recurrence had no evidence of generalized metastatic disease.

The cause of death in each of the 254 who have died is interesting. Only 53 in this series died of cancer of the prostate. In contrast to this relatively low figure among those who died without cancer, 97 died of cardiovascular disease. Eight died ultimately of respiratory failure. In 37, the pathologist could not find a definite cause of death. The cause of death in 33 others was listed "unknown".

The largest number of patients presented here in five year periods, lie in the 60 to 64 age group. The average age is 65.6. (Fig. 1).

We have gathered our patients into age groups and by presenting these figures for visual comparison with the U. S. Bureau of Vital Statistics' curve of anticipated length of life for these same age groups, we believe we are showing a more accurate measure of comparative survival. The more frequently presented method of survival statistics is by comparison of the operated group's average age at the time of operation with the mortality statistics of the total U.S.A. male population between 50 and 75 years of age. This "linear" statistical calculation in Figure 2 presents a 5 year survival figure of 71.8 %, a 10 year survival period of 38.6 % and a 15 year survival period of 21.6 % for our patients.

Figure 3 reveals the more accurate story by showing the survival in 5 year periods of the group under consideration as compared to the life expectancy of American males in the same 5 year groups. In these figures the time of survival in years is checked off on the ordinate, patient ages in the abscissa. The life expectancy of the U.S.A. males in 1959 to 1961 is marked "0". In Figure 3 the curve for 398 patients

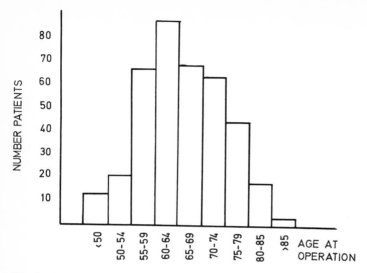

Fig. 1. Age distribution in five year groups of 398 patients who underwent total perineal prostatectomy for cancer of the prostate.

Years followed	Numer of Patients	Number of Patients survived	Number Survivors in %
5	398	285	71.8
10	303	117	38.6
15	218	47	21.6

Fig. 2. Five, ten and fifteen year survival in a group of 398 patients who underwent total perineal prostatectomy prior to 1965.
Average age 65.6 years, oldest 86 years, youngest 46 years.

operated prior to 1965 is marked with one dot. The curve of 303 patients operated prior to 1960 is marked with two dots and the curve of 218 patients operated prior to 1955 is marked with three dots. Thus one dot represents a 5 to 10 year follow-up, two dots 10 to 15 years and three dots a 15 year and more follow-up thus relating patient-age at operation to life expectancy. Viewing this chart it is apparent that there is no marked difference between the different groups. It shows also that

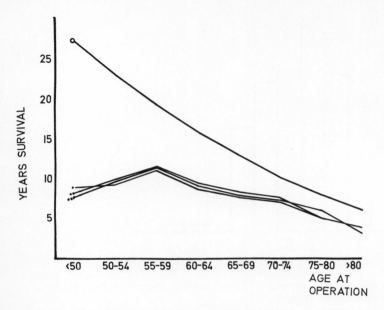

Fig. 3. The line ○ represents the average life expectancy of the USA male.
The line ● represents the average years of survival after operation of 398 patients operated upon prior to 1965 constituting a five to ten year follow-up.
The line ● ● represents the average years of survival of 308 patients operated upon prior to 1960; a ten to fifteen year follow-up.
The line ● ● ● represents the average years of survival of 218 patients operated upon prior to 1955; a follow-up of 15 years and longer.

the best life expectancy lies in the 55 to 59 year old age group and the least life expectancy in the younger group between 50 and 54 years of age. This is to be compared to the usually recorded life expectancy for a man of this age group. Thus a glimpse of the natural history of this disease is afforded by the demonstration in this curve of the greater severity of cancer of the prostate in the younger age group.

In Figure 4 we have pulled apart the dead from the living, the dead being represented in the two dot line and the living in the three dot line. This is to be compared to the overall survival rate in the one dot line and all three are comparable to the true survival rate for the American male as demonstrated in the line marked by "0". The figure seems to show that the nearest to the normal survival rate is attained in the 70 to 80 age group. These latter are the tough old survivors of all of the storms of human life. They number 30 in this study.

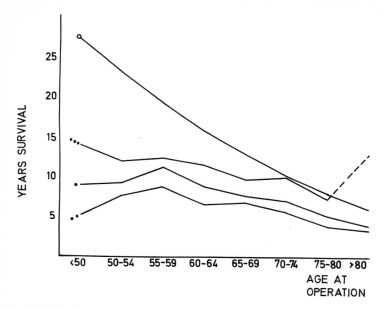

Fig. 4. The line ○ represents the life expectancy of the USA male.

The line ● represents the average years of survival after operation by five year periods of our entire group of 398 patients.

The line ● ● represents the average years of survival after surgery of those who have died.

The line ● ● ● represents the average years of survival after operation of those who are still living.

In Figure 5 we are demonstrating years of survival in relation to extension beyond the capsule. Line "0" again represents the life expectancy of the U.S.A. male, 1959 to 1961, and is given for comparison. Dot one, presents the average survival of the whole series in age groups. Dots two, the 166 patients in whom the disease had not extended through the capsule and dots three, the 288 patients in whom the pathologist found microscopic extension through the prostatic capsule or into the seminal vesicles. The figure shows the considerable spread in these mortality figures. The brief life span of those patients in whom the disease had spread beyond the capsule is evident.

Figure 6 shows a much closer relationship of the three lines under study and represents the years of survival in relation to the grade of lesion, demonstrating the apparently small importance of grade in relation to survival; however, grading in 89 of our patients was not carried out, reducing by this number the value of this information.

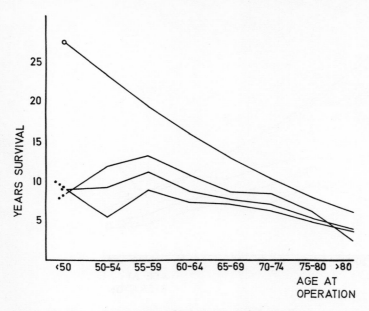

Fig. 5. The line ○ represents the life expectancy of the USA male.

The line ● represents the average years of survival after operation by five year periods of our entire group of 398 patients.

The line ● ● represents the average years of survival after operation of 170 patients who had no microscopic extension of cancer beyond the prostatic capsule.

The line ● ● ● represents the average years of survival after operation of 228 patients who had microscopic extension of their prostatic cancer beyond the prostatic capsule or into the seminal vesicles.

Figure 7 compares the survival rate of the entire series represented in the one dot line to the two dot line which shows the years of survival in the 53 patients who had tumor dissemination as metastases throughout the body and who died of carcinoma of the prostate with metastases. The degree of malignancy of prostatic carcinoma in the aged is demonstrated in this study by the fact that there were 5 patients operated upon in the 75 to 80 group who, in spite of a total prostatectomy in a seemingly confined prostate, died of multiple metastases. The time of survival of these patients was relatively long in comparison to the total 398 patients.

Another surprising revelation is that the time of survival of the 16 patients having multiple metastases in the age group between 50 and 59 approximates the length of the survival time of the total group. The years of survival of these 16 patients with obviously extremely malignant prostatic disease averaged 9 years; greatest 15 years, least 1 year.

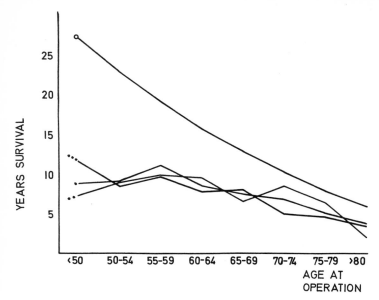

Fig. 6. The line ○ represents the life expectancy of the USA male.

The line ● represents the average years of survival after operation in five year groups of our entire series of 398 patients.

The line ● ● represents the average years of survival of 149 patients who had Grades I and II prostatic cancers.

The line ● ● ● represents the average years of survival of 108 patients who had Grades III and IV prostatic cancer.

In conclusion our statistical study of 398 patients upon whom we performed total perineal prostatectomy for prostatic cancer is presented grouped in five year periods of survival after the initial surgery. In our tables and figures direct comparison of our patient survival rates in 5 year periods with the survival rates of the average United States male by age groups is readily possible. It is seen that averaging all patients considered here the life expectance after surgery of this group of patients is approximately half of the national life expectancy in each age group. It is clear also that in the younger decade, 50 to 59, the life expectancy is considerably less than in the advanced age groups. This disturbingly higher mortality in the younger age groups is not the result of a greater incidence of cancer recurrence but is apparently due to other incidental illnesses, especially heart disease; indicating a greater frailty in this particular group of males. This higher incidence of cancer

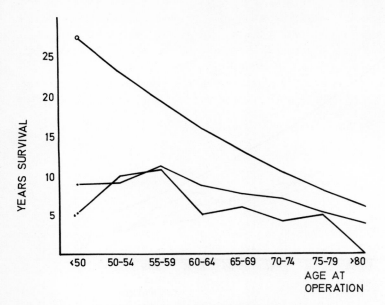

Fig. 7. The line ○ represents the life expectancy of the USA male.

The line ● represents the average years of survival after operation in five year groups of our entire series of 398 patients.

The line ● ● represents the average survival time of the 53 patients in this series who died of prostatic cancer with metastases.

mortality is in accord with the general opinion that prostatic cancer is thought to be a more virulent disease in younger than in older men. The question, however, remains: Why do so large a proportion of these young males in this series die early in spite of being free of cancer? In this entire group of 398 patients, 53 patients died from metastatic disease, or 12.5 %. In contrast, in the age group below 50, 7 of 13 patients died of metastases, making 53.8 %.

A thoughtful consideration of the statistics presented in this brief review comprising a study of the ultimate fate of 398 patients with carcinoma of the prostate after total perineal prostatectomy must lead to the conclusion that, early or late, and the grade not withstanding, carcinoma of the prostate is by no means a mild and harmless disease.

Not shown here in this cold consideration of life expectancy alone is the outstanding fact that after the total removal of the prostate, the site of origin in this type of cancer, life is more tolerable. There seldom is local recurrence. Distant metastases seldom produce intolerable pain but are controllable chemically with drugs and hormones. Cobalt treatment also plays a helpful role when cancer recurrs. Urinary infection rarely occurs and is always readily controlled when the bladder neck remains widely open as it does in perineal prostatectomy patients.

The prostatic cancer patient, selected for total perineal prostatectomy, has a much greater chance of long life than has the prostatic cancer patient treated by any other means.

Discussion

W. E. Goodwin: I am going first to call on Dr. *Veenema.* In our program we have heard about total perineal prostatectomy from Dr. *Belt* but we have not heard the answer to the question which was asked yesterday by Prof. *Alken,* as to what do we think about radical retropubic prostatectomy. So, Dr. *Ralph Veenema,* from Columbia University, will you please speak on the subject of retropubic prostatectomy.

R. J. Veenema: At Columbia-Presbyterian since 1951 we have done mainly radical retropubic prostatectomy or as Dr. *Belt* says, the total prostato vesiculectomy. From 1951 to 1967 there were 144 patients who underwent the total prostatectomy, and a recent review of those with at least 9 year follow-up shows a survival of 73 %. Interestingly, this parallels many of the other series as well. The one reason that we have done the radical retropubic is that we chose to do our biopsy by the"perineal-cup"method and if the lesion is in the operable phase, i.e.,stages 1 and 2, we will proceed with the total retropubic prostatectomy. The functional result following this total removal shows 10 % of patients are incontinent and wear a device. All of the patients are impotent. The majority of the patients had a bilateral orchiectomy at the same time as the radical retropubic prostatectomy. There were 5 patients who had delayed radical retropubics. 4 of those are living – 12, 11, 9 and 6 years later. By delayed radical prostatectomy we mean those who were in between an operable and an inoperable phase. Thus orchiectomy was done and the patients then became more suitable for surgery, usually within a 3-6 month period.

W. Brosig: I think the German colleagues would like to know what are the exact indications for radical prostatectomy? Up to now we have not operated on patients who are older than 70. Now, we have seen some of Dr. *Belt's* cases who are much older.

The other question is – if you have done a radical prostatectomy, should you also do oestrogen therapy? In some cases they do, in some cases they do not. In what cases should you do it?

The third question I would like to ask is – what is the advantage of retropubic, compared to perineal prostatectomy? Which method is better? Which method should you do?

J. J. Kaufman: I did not come prepared to discuss the relative merits of perineal and radical retropubic prostatectomy, but Prof. *Alken* asked me to discuss some of the areas of apparent controversy in our own thinking about radical prostatectomy and some of the other modalities in the treatment of carcinoma of the prostate in the United States. What shall we advise our German colleages if they are about to embark on a program of radical surgery for operable carcinoma of the prostate? Well as you know, and as you have heard, there are 2 schools in America – the perineal school and the retropubic school. I would say, that I think that for people who are starting to do radical prostatectomy the retropubic approach is probably better. Dr. *Belt* is an expert in perineal surgery. He has fantastic experience. The rest of us who have been trained in perineal surgery, and I was trained almost 20 years ago by Dr. *Goodwin,* also do perineal surgery, but we do not do it quite so well, and quite so expeditiously. I personally am turning towards retropubic prostatectomy, for several reasons.

I think this approach is one that we use a great deal more. We are familiar with the retropubic area, as a result of doing cystectomies, as a result of doing YV plasties on the bladder neck, as a result of doing more retropubic "simple" prostatectomies. The perineum is familiar to us, but not as familiar as the retropubic area. The disadvantages of the retropubic prostatectomy are that you must rely on a needle biopsy, or a "cup" biopsy, whereas with the perineal approach you can have a more definitive biopsy by the open technique. However, with experience and with the use of the precautions that I mentioned yesterday about using "good" instruments, new needles, one can be very accurate in taking samples of prostatic tissue through the perineum with a needle. As far as the anastamosis between the bladder neck and the urethra is concerned, there is no question that this is probably better via the perineal approach than by the retropubic approach.

As far as control of bleeding is concerned, perhaps there is about a 50/50 division between the ease of handling the pedicle by the perineal approach and the retropubic approach. Bleeding is perhaps a little less by the perineal approach than by the retropubic approach. However, using the perineal route haemorrhoids have occurred more often in the post operative period. This is not a problem with the retropubic approach.

As far as morbidity and mortality for the patient is concerned – I think mortality rate must be considered to be lower by the perineal than by the retropubic approach. Patients tolerate the perineal approach extremely well. There seems to be an equal morbidity in terms of impotence and incontinence in the 2 operations, although I do not think that that is any bone of contention.

The retropubic approach does allow exposure of the iliac vessels, so that you can detect early metastases – a point that has been alluded too by Dr. *Flocks.* He has stated, and it has been confirmed by others, that 10 % of patients with early lesions of the prostate will have lymph node metastases. Does it help to know about these metastases? In other words, if we were to combine a radical iliac lymph node dissection with a radical prostatectomy – would it materially aid in the prognosis? I do not think anyone can tell us that and probably it is just some knowledge that we can put to use in our subsequent decision as to whether we use oestrogen or orchiectomy in these patients.

Our own feeling at the present time about orchiectomy and oestrogen is that we reserve these for patients who have symptomatic metastases. We do not use them prophylactically.

Well in summary, I would say that there are a number of experienced perineal surgeons such as Dr. *Whitmore,* who have converted recently to the radical retropubic approach. I am dividing my operations between the two, chiefly because I feel that I want to keep my familiarity with the perineum, and at the same time build up my own expertise with the radical retropubic approach. I hope that this has answered some of your questions. As you can see, this is an arbitrary matter, but the perineal school is a very esoteric school. Very much like the cold punch resectionists who are excellent in their particular line, from having been trained at the Mayo clinic in this technique, but for the *rest* of us it is something that we can admire but *not* participate in. So I would say that those of you who are embarking upon a program and have *not* been trained in perineal surgery – the retropubic approach is probably the one that I would advise you to perfect.

W. E. Goodwin: If the moderator may be permitted to comment on what Dr. *Kaufman* has just said — I have to quote *Hugh Young,* who said that the Lord intended for the prostate to be approached from the perineum, that is why he put it so close to the outside at that point.

R. Übelhör*: As to the questions of Prof. *Brosig:*

Few carcinomas of the prostate can be classified as operable at the time of diagnosis. After several months of oestrogen therapy, however, some of them become smaller and better delineated to such an extent that one might consider the tumor operable.

One may assume that in the case of a positive response to oestrogen therapy after removal of the primary tumor the surrounding tissue which is still infiltrated by cancerous tissue can be better controlled than if the tumor is present. There is some clinical evidence indicating that *Huggin's* statement, "Cancer is safest when completely removed and preserved in pickel" is also true for those carcinomas which originally appeared to be inoperable.

If the presence of carcinoma can be proved by needle-biopsy and metastases excluded, oestrogen therapy should be immediately started after irradiation of the mammal gland in order to avoid gynecomastia. 3 to 6 months later prostatectomy together with orchidectomy should be performed. Orchidectomy is advisable because the recommended continuation of oestrogen therapy is all too often interrupted by the patient if he feels well. Subsequently there should be a low-dosed oral longterm therapy.

Vasico-urethral anastomosis

I prefer the retropubic access. In my opinion a particularly weak point in the usual technique is that a tension-free connection between the bladder and the urethra is not possible. Many years ago *Flocks* proposed the formation of a tube out of a flap from the anterior bladder wall to be interposed between the bladder and urethra. Unaware of this publication I have tried the same technique and five years ago published. The remarkable feature is the complete continence from the very beginning and only a low tendency towards stricture.

Technique

Low abdominal median laparotomy. Transverse incision of the anterior wall of the empty bladder immediately above the palpable margin of the prostate. Insertion of two ureter catheters which remain for ten days. Completion of the anterior incision to a circular one and separation of the bladder from the prostate. Clamping and lifting of the posterior bladder wall and blunt separation of the bladder from the vesicular glands. After reaching the upper end of the vesicular glands and after dissection of the deferent ducts, the prerectal space is prepared. The prostate and vesicular glands are clamped in toto and the separation from the rectum is performed with the aid of cranial-ventral traction. The vessels on both sides are now ligated.

Dissection of the apex of the prostrate from the urethra. With this, prostatectomy is completed.

Formation of a 4 cm-wide and 7 cm-long flap from the anterior bladder wall.

If a completely tension-free anastomosis between the tube and the urethra is not possible, better mobilisation of the bladder can be achieved by extraperitonealisation. Formation of a tube out of the bladder flap by means of a two-layer interrupted suture (mucosa: 4-zero chromic catgut, outer layer: 2-zero chromic catgut). A U-tube FG 16 or 18 with lateral holes is inserted. The cranial end of the U-tube and the ureter catheters are led out suprapubically far from

* Director, Urolog. Universitätsklinik, Wien, Austria.

the base of the newly formed tube. The closure of the bladder in a horizontal line is achieved by means of fixation sutures. The other end of the U-tube is led out through the urethra, and the anastomosis of the tube to the urethra is performed by a total of 4 to 6 interrupted single-layer 2-zero chromic catgut sutures.

H. Marberger: I would like to make one comment on surgical treatment of prostatic cancer. When we looked up our results in a series of 350 cases, we were struck by one fact. If you follow up prostatic carcinoma cases with supra – vesicular obstruction, you see that 30 % of them die in the first year and 40 % are dead after two years. Now if you compare these figures with carcinoma of all kinds, even with metastases, without obstruction of the ureters, you see that the percentage of mortality in the first two years is 6 % and 18 %. So we studied these cases more carefully and we found out that about half of them die, not due to cancer, but due to a secondary urological complication. I think that in filghting the cancer we should not forget to do things we normally do in our daily urological practice.

Posterior capsule

R. T. Turner–Warwick: I wish to discuss the problem of the posterior capsule. We, for many years, in my unit, have used this technique, to make an excision of the posterior capsule – full thickness – the whole of this. In other words, having made the enucleation, to remove separately the whole of this. We do not do this as a prophylactic treatment, although possibly sooner or later one could remove some focus which is important. We do it because it is a diagnostic "extra" for the patient who has a "normal-feeling" posterior capsule. We sometimes do it as an excisional biopsy of a "hard" nodule in the posterior capsule. It is very easy to do this resection as you shall see, and then you can do a frozen section, and proceed to a radical retropubic, if you wish. We do it sometimes, of course, as a curative procedure when you have chronic infection in the posterior capsule and in the vesicles. We, actually, prefer to do it as a routine, because it makes a neat urethral reconstruction with re-epithelialisation. If the biopsy is negative, well then of course, you discharge the patient. If the biopsy is positive (you have evidence of microscopic tumour), well then, of course, you have a problem. I am not going to discuss the problem, so much as just to make the comment on the method of getting the histology.

Intra- and postoperative problems

E. Belt: In our own work we definitely feel that we can prevent blood loss to a greater extent using perineal prostatectomy than we can with total retropubic prostatectomy. The anastamosis of the urethra to the bladder neck after the prostate has been completely removed can also be achieved perineally. An end to end anastamosis can be done, because the operation is under complete visual control throughout. You see what you are doing.

It is a disadvantage to discover that there is no lymph node involvement. I suppose that not being able to see lymph node involvement and then to discontinue the operation is a disadvantage. Knowledge of such involvement could possibly cut down postoperative recurrences.

Recently we have also been using strontium scans, and our figures are not 10 %, but 25 %. These are people in whom we have found no evidence of extension with the conventional methods (X–Ray and so on), who on strontium scan reveal bone extension. Recently we had a man who came all the way from Brazil to us for total prostatectomy because his urologist had found that he was free of metastases. We did a strontium bone scan and sent him all the way back home again, because his bone scan showed great areas of bone involvement with cancer.

Our experience with sexual power after total prostatectomy is very interesting, in that 10 % of our patients retain their sexual power and a few of them have – well, their wives have complained to me about this – that they seem never to get through sexual intercourse and want to repeat it so often that it becomes wearisome to the wife. I don't know what brings this about. If I did I'd like to patent it.

The other thing is incontinence. We have 10 % incontinence of urine, and I don't know what it is that causes this either, but it looks as if *Joe Kaufman* with his Kaufman"King's-X"operation has found a cure for that.

Total perineal prostatectomy (demonstration by film)

W. E. Goodwin: Next we will see a film on the technique of total perineal prostatectomy, presented by Dr. *Belt,* who will make some introductory remarks.

E. Belt: The position in perineal prostatectomy is important. The perineum is brought almost parallel to the floor by dipping the head end of the table downwards. The instruments we use are these: A simple sound, lateral retractors of several lengths, the prostatic tractor, and the posterior retractor. These special instruments are not necessary. Adequate instruments can be selected from any good surgical locker but these make things more convenient.

The first figure shows the curving incision made 1 1/2 cm above the mucocutaneous juncture (fig. 1a). In the dissection of the perineum, the frenulum, which runs along the under surface of the penis, over the scrotum, down to the rectum, is a median raphe. It is recognized by pulling downward on the skin flap. It is identified and incised. Then the rectal sphincters are elevated by blunt dissection (fig. 1b). The sphincters surround the anal ring and can be lifted right off the anterior fascia of the rectum sweeping them upward with the handle of the scalpel. Thus the apex of the prostate is revealed. The levator ani are then pushed laterally thus revealing the entire posterior aspect of the prostate (fig. 1c).

If a benign adenoma of the prostate is to be removed the prostatic capsule is entered distal to the verumontanum. This area can be located by the pressure of the index finger against a sound which at this point is placed through the urethra into the bladder and serves to press the prostate backward into the operative field holding it firmly in position as the dissection proceeds. It is by finger dissection that a benign adenoma is separated from the prostatic capsule. The finger follows the cleavage plane between the adenoma and the prostatic capsule. Great care is taken not to tear the membranous urethra. It is clearly revealed by careful dissection and then cleanly cut across with scissors leaving a clearly defined tube of urethra which can later be precisely anastomosed to the circular bladder neck with precisely placed sutures under direct vision.

This is the singular great advantage of perineal prostatectomy for both benign adenectomy and total prostatectomy for cancer. In no other method of prostatic removal is the continuity of the urethra precisely restored.

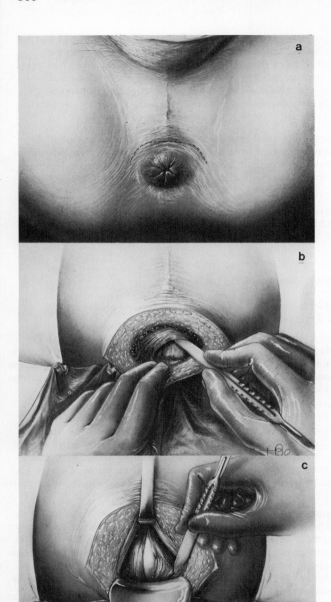

Fig. 1a–c

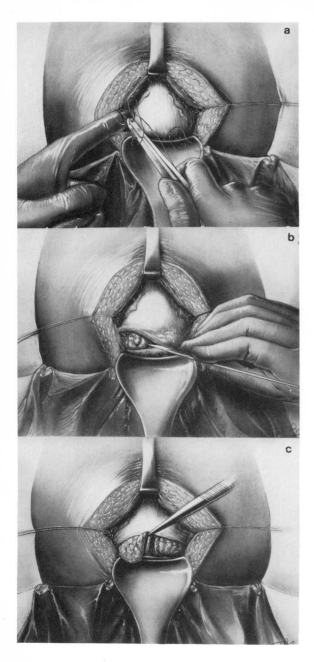

Fig. 2a−c

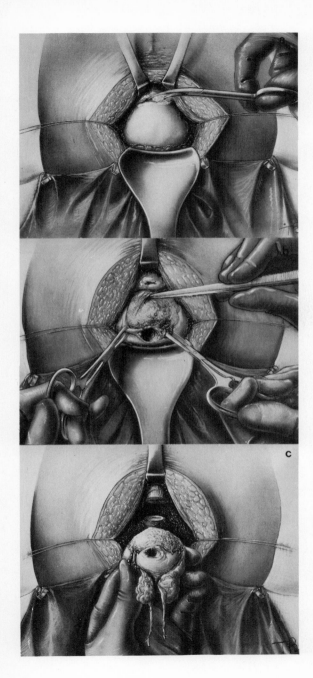

Fig. 3a–c

If the surgery is to be total removal of the prostate for cancer, the capsule is not opened. The blood supply of the prostate coming into it posteriorly from each side is easily recognized, clamped, cut and ligated, (fig. 2a). Denonvilliers' fascia is then incised transversely close to the base of the prostate to gain access to the seminal vesicles (fig. 2b). Each seminal vesical is dissected from its bed together with the ampullae of each vas deferens (fig. 2c). The large blood vessel which enters each seminal vesicle at its apex is carefully ligated. A long strip of vas is dissected from the retrovesical tissue to be removed with the specimen.

Turning then to the apex of the prostate the membranous urethra is cut across as close to the prostatic tissue as possible (fig. 3a). This dissection is carried forward between the anterior aspect of the prostatic capsule and the rich plexi of veins which cling to it (fig. 3b). These veins are not disturbed. The prostate now remains attached to the bladder by the urethra and its mucosa at the bladder neck. This tube of mucosa is cut across with scissors and the prostate with capsule, both seminal vesicles and both ampullae and a long section of each vas is lifted from the wound (fig. 3c).

Careful anastomosis of the bladder neck to the urethra is effected around a catheter carrying a 30 cc bulb. The first of four stitches is placed anteriorly while a urethral catheter which has been pushed through the urethra is elevated lifting the cutoff end of the urethra into the field of vision (fig. 4a). The urethral catheter is then inserted into the bladder. The tube of mucosa which forms

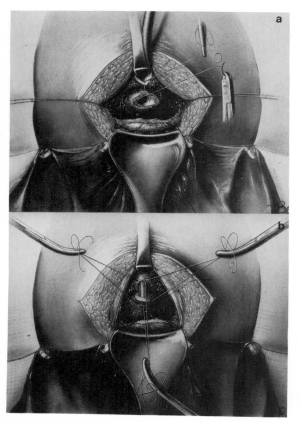

Fig. 4a—b

the bladder neck and the tube of urethral mucosa formerly at the apex of the prostate approximate one another along this catheter. Two lateral stitches and one posterior stitch in these structures effect an anastomosis between them (fig. 4b).

The thin layer of Denonvilliers' fascia which covered the seminal vesicles and was incised transversely over them is now lifted up and stitched to the adventitia which envelopes the membranous urethra (fig. 5a). This layer of fascia gives additional support to the anastomosis between the urethra and the bladder neck. It adds one more cover or layer to the urethra helping to insure per primum healing (fig. 5b).

The levator ani muscles are now brought together with interrupted stitches. Number 00 chromic catgut is used throughout. The wound is closed in layers. The skin is closed with a running subcuticular stitch. A drain which has been left in place is taken out the next morning. Each day the wound is baked with an infrared lamp twice, 20 minutes at a time. We have per primum healing.

Surgical mortality is very low. It is perhaps 1 %. I think we have had 3 surgical deaths in 400 cases.

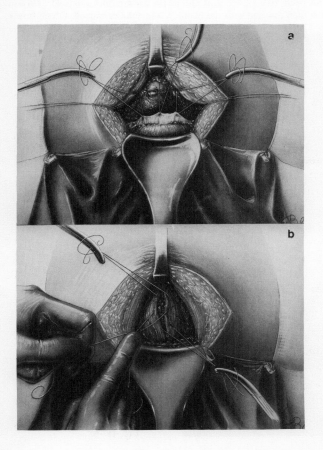

Fig. 5a—b

Modern Radiotherapy of Prostatic Cancer

M. A. Bagshaw

Division of Radiation Therapy, Stanford University School of Medicine, Stanford, California 94305, USA

Summary: The advent of modern megavoltage radiotherapy devices such as ^{60}CO units, linear accelerators, and betatrons has stimulated radiotherapists to explore their potential usefulness in the treatment of certain neoplasms not usually considered radiocurable. One of these is carcinoma of the prostate which because it remains reasonably localized for long periods of time within a relatively small volume of tissue represents an ideal situation for radiation therapy. During the past 13 years 308 patients with localized carcinoma of the prostate have been irradiated by means of the Stanford Medical Linear Accelerator. A tumor dose of approximately 7,500 rads homogeneously distributed within a cylindrical volume of tissue 6 cm in diameter and 6 cm in height fractionated over a period of seven weeks has been used in most cases. Survival rates of 58 % at five years and 40 % at ten years have been observed. While this technique may not replace radical prostatectomy in the patient with a well circumscribed small nodule as the treatment of choice, it does offer an alternate method of definitive treatment for patients with neoplasm too extensive for radical resection but still localized to the region of the prostate, periprostatic tissue, and seminal vesicles.

The rapid development of megavoltage techniques in radiotherapy during the past 20 years has stimulated renewed interest in the radiotherapy of carcinoma of the prostate, one of the most common forms of cancer in the male [1—4].

Before proceeding with a discussion of the more than 300 patients who have been treated by external megavoltage radiation therapy at Stanford University since 1956, it is of interest to review briefly the milestones in the treatment of prostatic cancer in an attempt to understand why the application of radiation therapy in this disease has been neglected for so long. The first definitive approach to the treatment of prostatic cancer was introduced by *Young* [5] in 1904 with the description of his classic operation, the radical perineal prostatectomy. Although this procedure has proven effective in some cases, it was appreciated that the key to its success was dependent upon the proper selection of patients. Thus, nearly 70 years after the introduction of radical perineal prostatectomy we find its advocates becoming increasingly rigid in their criteria of operability. It is not surprising, therefore, that the *Young* School of Urology soon looked to other methods of therapy and introduced

Manuscript received: 14 November 1969

in the 1920's the treatment of prostatic cancer by the insertion of a radium source into the lumen of the prostatic urethra. Thus, in 1922 and 1924 publications describing this method appeared [6, 7]. Following this, radiotherapists of the 1930's were attempting to treat prostatic cancer by means of teletherapy in the range of 180–220 KeV. For example, *Bernard Widmann* [8] in 1934 reported excellent palliation in a group of patients treated by this type of irradiation. His patients were grossly advanced and debilitated because of symptoms of pain and urinary obstruction. In spite of their advanced status and the limitations of his radiotherapeutic equipment, he was able to achieve remarkable palliation and objective tumor remission, therefore, demonstrating that this usually well differentiated adenocarcinoma is in fact radioresponsive. These early indications of the possible radiocurability of prostatic cancer probably would have received more attention had it not been for the demonstration of hormone dependency in malignant disease. Hormone manipulation either by the administration of estrogens or castration became widely accepted for nearly all patients with prostatic cancer except those with extremely localized disease who might still be treated definitively by radical surgery.

The application of irradiation achieved renewed significance in 1951 when Dr. *Flocks* [9] introduced the interstitial injection of a solution of radioactive gold [198]Au colloid directly into the prostate. Subsequent modifications of this technique and results will be presented by Dr. *Flocks*.

Quite independently in the mid – 1950's several authors started to reexamine the application of external beam therapy in the treatment of primary prostatic cancer, particularly in view of the greatly improved radiation techniques made possible by megavoltage equipment [1–4].

At Stanford a small travelling-wave linear accelerator was designed and fabricated in 1955 for the production of a 5 MEV X-ray beam which could be well collimated and which could be used as a general radiation source for radiotherapy. This was the first unit of its kind in the United States and soon after its introduction we were asked to treat a patient with prostatic cancer. One could trace the origin of our interest to the much earlier work stemming from the use of an intra-catheter radium source. Dr. *James Ownby,* our urological consultant was familiar with the old Hopkins' radium technique and indeed had used this method in the treatment of one of his patients. Three years following treatment the patient again developed obstructive symptoms due to regrowth of the carcinoma and he requested that we consider re-irradiation by means of the linear accelerator. We were familiar with the recent work of Dr. *Flocks* and decided that his demonstration of the radioresponsiveness to interstitial irradiation with [198]Au colloid was sufficient precedent to utilize the linear accelerator in the treatment of this disease.

1. Patient selection

In selecting patients for the investigation of definitive radiotherapy, the following criteria must be met.

(1) The diagnosis must be proven by biopsy. In most instances this is accomplished by a simple transrectal needle biopsy. In the event of failure, a transperineal needle biopsy is attempted. If a transurethral resection is necessary to establish the diagnosis, it usually indicates that the patient has somewhat more extensive disease and that function of the prostatic urethra and bladder has already been compromised by obstruction and/or infection. Although we believe that this is the least optimum method for proving the diagnosis, there are instances when the transurethral approach is necessary in order to relieve the patient's acute symptoms.

(2) While patients with locally advanced disease, i.e., involvement of the prostatic capsule or seminal vesicles are acceptable for therapy, patients with metastatic disease are not included in this series. This does not mean that patients with metastatic disease may not benefit from irradiation of the primary lesion when the primary lesion is symptomatic; we simply have not included patients with metastatic disease which was known prior to the institution of therapy in this group. The search for metastatic disease includes X-ray films of the axial skeleton, chest X-ray, acid and alkaline phosphatase determinations, and in selected instances, a ^{85}Sr bone scan. We have not accepted the elevation of the acid phosphatase as a sole criterium for rejection of a patient for treatment, however, it is useful for supplementary evidence of metastatic disease in instances where the scintiscan or X-ray examination is equivocal. Finally, although we have tended to accept patients whose local disease is somewhat too advanced for consideration of radical perineal prostatectomy, we have accepted patients for treatment with solitary nodular prostatic cancer when the patient has refused more definitive surgical resection. This has occurred in a number of incidences in relatively young individuals who are unwilling to accept the almost certain impotence which follows the radical perineal operation.

2. Stanford technique

In the Stanford technique the patient is treated in the standing position (Fig. 1). The platform upon which the patient stands is adjustable along an X- and Y-axis so that the position of the prostate may be carefully situated along the central axis of the treatment beam. Thus, when the patient is rotated through either a 360° arc or two lateral 120° arcs, the prostate is at the dead center of rotation and the radiation dose is homogeneous and concentrated (Fig. 2 and 3). The urinary bladder lies superior to the treatment field, the testes are inferior to the treatment field and are not irradiated.

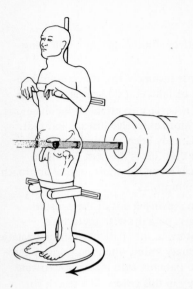

Fig. 1
The patient is treated standing, resting upon a rotational platform that is capable of either 360° rotation or rotation through any segment of a 360° arc.

PROSTATE or BLADDER

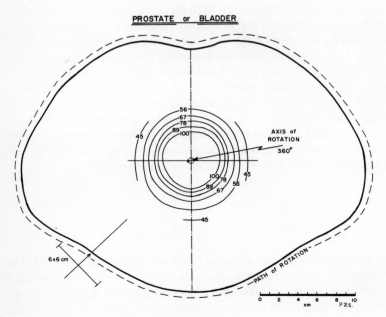

Fig. 2. Isodose contour for 360° rotation with a 6 × 6 cm field. The field dimensions are measured at the axis of rotation. Note that the dose to the prostate region is entirely homogeneous, that is, lies within the 100 % line.

By using the lateral 120° arcs, the dose distribution is extended laterally along the natural lines of fixation of the prostate to the pelvic sidewall. We try to achieve a maximum dose of 7,500 rads at the isocenter over a period of about 7 weeks. In order to accomplish this we believe that the irradiated volume must be kept to a minimum. Therefore, we employ a localization technique which permits visualization of the prostatic urethra by the introduction of a Foley catheter into the bladder. The bag of the Foley catheter is filled with mercury, a small amount of renographin contrast material is introduced into the bladder itself and a small amount of barium solution is introduced into the rectum (Fig. 4). With these organs opacified and with visulization of the prostatic urethra it is possible to localize accurately the position of the prostate and to direct the X-ray beam accordingly. A verification portal film is presented in Figure 5. Since the amount of periprostatic tissue which may be irradiated to a relatively high dose can be controlled by the appropriate selection of the field size, we need not select patients in whom the neoplasm is strictly confined to the prostate. But we may also treat patients who have involvement of the capsule, the seminal vesicles, or the immediately adjacent periprostatic tissue.

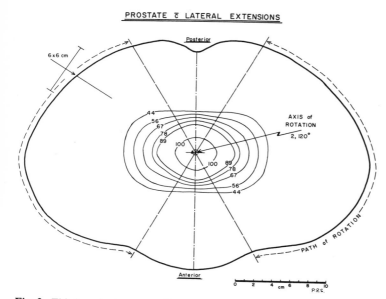

Fig. 3. This is an isodose curve for the dose distribution of radiation when left and right lateral arcs of 120° are used. Notice that the isodose curves extend laterally and that the region of interest lies within the 89 % isodose contour. This technique is especially useful when there is lateral extension of the neoplasm toward the pelvic sidewalls.

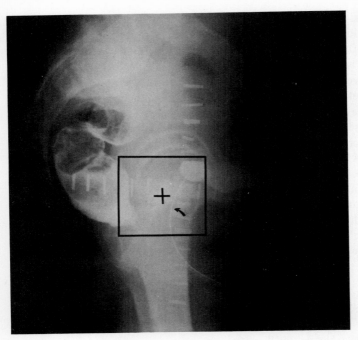

Fig. 4. A lateral roentgenogram which demonstrates the position of the prostate by virtue of which has been filled with mercury. Renographin is also instilled in the urinary bladder and opacification of the prostatic wether with a Foley catheter, the ballon of barium in the rectum in order to further delineate the position of the prostate. The black square demonstrates the position of the radiation volume. The black cross the central axis of the treatment beam.

3. Results

There have been 308 patients treated by this method between December 1956 and 1 January 1969. The overall survival is presented as a cumulative survival curve in Figure 6. One notices that at 5 years 58 % of the patients are surviving and at 10 years 40 % are surviving. Beyond 10 years 32 % survive but the numbers of patients entered into the study at 11, 12, and 13 years are relatively small. Even so, a 32 % survival at 13 years is quite acceptable when one considers that the mean age at the time of therapy was 67. While at 5 years the survival percentages are not much different than those reported for estrogen therapy, it should be remembered that a significant percentage of patients presented herein have had their primary neoplasm completely destroyed by irradiation. Thus, it would be expected that a relatively high level of

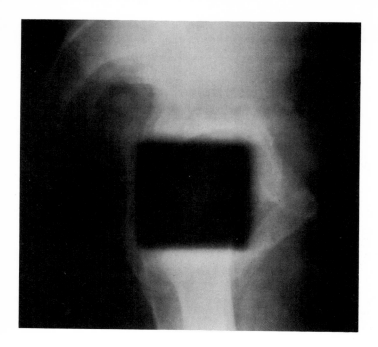

Fig. 5. Portal film which confirms the localization film presented in Figure 4. This is a double exposure roentgenogram, the blackened area in the prostatic region was produced by the treatment beam from the linear accelerator.

survival would be observed at 10 years. In a more detailed review of the first 150 cases reported here, the survival was 80 % at 5 years and 71 % at 10 years for 80 patients with nodular carcinoma confined to the prostate, 54 % at both 5 and 10 years in 50 patients with the entire gland involved and 24 % at 5 and 10 years in 16 patients with extension beyond the prostate either into the seminal vesicles or extending to the pelvic sidewalls.

Figure 7 demonstrates the survival in patients who had not received concomitant hormone manipulation as opposed to those who had received concomitant hormone treatment. Included in this sample are the first 137 consecutive patients treated. It was our policy to advise our referring urologists to discontinue estrogen therapy in order to permit the evaluation of the value of radiation alone. In some instances our colleagues would not accept this recommendation and therefore estrogen therapy

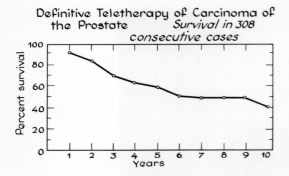

Fig. 6

Overall survival curve of patients treated with external irradiation for carcinoma of the prostate.

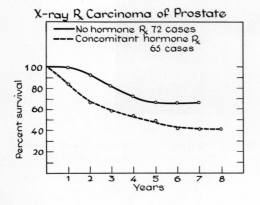

Fig. 7

Comparison of survival in patients who received concomitant hormone treatment with those receiving radiation therapy alone. See text for details.

was continued. In other instances orchiectomy had already been carried out prior to the referral of the patient and therefore it was impossible to reverse the patient's status. One notes a difference in survival, for example, at 7 years slightly more than 60 % of 72 patients were surviving who had received no hormone while at 7 years there was slightly more than 40 % survival in 65 cases who had received concomitant hormone therapy. In interpreting these data, however, one cannot conclude that the hormone treatment was detrimental since on the average, the extent of the disease at the time of therapy was more advanced in those patients who had already been previously Committed to hormone treatment.

In general, the response of prostatic neoplasm to irradiation as determined by digital examination is relatively slow. While shrinkage of the tumor during therapy is often noted, frequently there is little, if any, appreciable change at the conclusion of treatment. Periodic examinations, however, disclose the gradual reduction in size of the neoplasm, as well as the non-neoplastic portions of the prostate gland. By the time several months following therapy have elapsed an appreciable diminution in size is usually appreciated. In some patients with quite advanced disease, however, very little change is ever appreciated, although the nodularity may gradually change to simply persistent induration without much change in overall size. On the other hand, in patients who have complete regression of the tumor and who are followed for many years there is a gradual diminution in size of the prostate gland so that by 10 years, for example, there may be practically no prostatic tissue which can be appreciated by digital examination.

Finally, if we look at the crude survival in the group of patients who were treated between 5 and 10 years ago and hence, all have been at risk for at least 5 years, 25 of 59 are living without evidence of disease. 15 of these 25 have never had endocrine therapy, 28 are dead with neoplasm and 6 are still living but developed evidence of bone metastases at sometime during the interval.

4. Complications

Because the irradiated volume is relatively small and because this volume is situated outside the abdomen, tolerance to treatment during the course of therapy is excellent. During the final two weeks a few patients complain of moderate dysuria and others experience rectal discomfort and tenesmus, however, both of these side effects are rare (Fig. 8). In less than 2 % of the patients late urethral stricture has occurred which required surgical intervention. In these instances, the patients had extensive disease and required transurethral catheter drainage throughout their period of treatment. 5 % of the patients have experienced moderate to severe rectal discomfort or painless bleeding for a number of months following therapy. On proctoscopic examination, either edematous or hemorrhagic rectal mucosa is found overlying the prostate or small ulcerations of the rectal mucosa have been identified. In general, the symptoms may often be alleviated by hydrocortisone enemas and the lesions in all instances have healed with time. In several cases, however, 12 to 24 months have been required.

Ulceration Anterior Rectal Wall [1]	10 Pts	5 %
Urinary Incontinence (All had TUR Prior to X-ray)	4 Pts	2 %

[1] Most patients relieved by hydrocortisone enemas
    No colostomies

Fig. 8. Carcinoma of prostate. Significant sequelae in 215 patients.

So far it has not been necessary to resort to surgical intervention such as colostomy except in situations where the treatment has failed to control the progression of neoplastic disease.

While the evaluation of potency is difficult in this group of males for psychological reasons and the normal effect of aging, it is our best estimate that only one out of four patients becomes impotent subsequent to therapy.

In the United States, *Whitmore, Flocks,* and *Jewett* [9–11] have each achieved excellent results following the radical resection of the prostate in well selected patients. However, they have each called attention to the relatively small percentage of patients with prostatic cancer who are truly candidates for the operation when the disease is first diagnosed. It is likely that only between 5 and 10 % of all patients with this disease would be considered candidates for definitive surgery. For example, in *Jewett's* excellent series of 28 of 86 patients living without evident disease from 15 to 24 years following resection of a solitary nodule, his rigid criteria for selection indicated that the operation was applicable in only 7.9 % of the patients examined. On the other hand, 40 to 50 % of the patients with prostatic cancer may have the disease confined to the prostatic region but too extensive to warrant serious consideration of surgery alone. In these patients one could consider an attempt at curative therapy either by the method of *Flocks*, which includes subtotal resection and infiltration of the tumor bed by radioactive gold colloid or by megavoltage external beam therapy. It is possible that the percentage of patients in whom these latter modes of treatment might be applied will increase. For example, recent data in the State of California has demonstrated that the incidence of localized prostatic cancer has increased from 49 % in the interval 1940 through 1949 to 57 % in the interval 1960 through 1964. During the same period of time the percentage of patients treated by surgery only decreased from 48 to 30 %, while the percentage of patients treated by surgery plus chemotherapy and/or hormone therapy rose from 29 to 42. These trends suggest to me that, on one hand, carcinoma of the prostate is being recognized more frequently while still in a localized stage, and on the other hand, surgeons are becoming increasingly critical in their selection of patients for surgical resection. Thus, it appears that the general physician is being more conscientious in his effort to detect carcinoma of the prostate in a localized stage. This happy state compliments the efforts of the radiotherapist who may now offer definitive, potentially curative treatment to a large group of patients who otherwise would be relegated to palliative treatment only.

References

[1] *Budhraja, S. N.* and *Anderson, J. C.* : An Assessment of the Value of Radiotherapy in the Management of Carcinoma of the Prostate, British Journal of Urology, 36, 535–540, 1964.

[2] *Bagshaw, A.* et al.: Linear Accelerator Supervoltage Radiotherapy, VII Carcinoma of the Prostate, Radiology, 85, 121–129, July, 1965.

[3] *George, F. W.* et al.: Cobalt-60 Telecurietherapy in the Definitive Treatment of Carcinoma of the Prostate: A Preliminary Report, The Journal of Urology, 93, 102–109, January, 1965.

[4] *Del Regato, J. A.* : Radiotherapy in the Conservative Treatment of Operable and Locally Inoperable Carcinoma of the Prostate, Radiology, 88, 761–766, April, 1967.

[5] *Young, H. H.* : The Early Diagnosis and Radical Cure of Carcinoma of the Prostate: Being a Study of 40 Cases and Presentation of a Radical Operation Which Was Carried Out in Four Cases. Bull. Johns Hopkins Hosp. 16, 315–321, 1905.

[6] *Barringer, B. S.:* Radium in the Treatment of Prostatic Carcinoma, Ann. Surg., 80, 881–884, December, 1924.

[7] *Deming, C. L.* : Results of 100 Cases of Cancer of the Prostate and Seminal Vesicles Treated with Radium, Surg., Gynec. & Obst., 34, 99–118, January, 1922.

[8] *Widmann, B. P.* : Cancer of the Prostate. The Results of Radium and Roentgen-Ray Treatment, Radiology, 22,153–159, February, 1934.

[9] *Flocks, R. H.* et al.: Treatment of Carcinoma of the Prostate by Interstitial Radiation with Radio-Active Gold (^{198}Au): A Preliminary Report, J. Urol., 68, 510–522, August, 1952.

[10] *Whitmore, W. F.* et al.: Experiences with Various Operative Procedures for the Total Excision of Prostatic Cancer, Cancer, 396–405, March-April, 1959.

[11] *Jewett, H. J.* et al.: The Palpable Nodule of Prostatic Cancer, JAMA, 203, 403–406, February, 1968.

Discussion

R. J. Veenema: Dr. *Bagshaw's* paper was certainly most enjoyable. I have had the privilege of working with Dr. *Robert Sagarman,* who is from their department, and with Dr. *Ruth Guttman* of the Dellafield Department of Radiotherapy. From 1961 to June 1968 we irradiated 34 patients for prostatic cancer. These were not patients that we were treating as primary therapy, such as is Dr. *Bagshaw's* main series. These were patients who were hormonally refractory, and had obstructive uropathy of varying degrees, with persistent or recurrent haematuria. The radiotherapy was used in an effort to increase pallation. I think our experience has added, to the evidence of the radio-sensitivity of the prostate.

The residual urine was improved in 14 of the 23 patients, who had a considerably elevated residual urine and recurrent infections. Haematuria was improved in all of those who had it, and ureteral obstruction, pelvic pain, lymphatic obstruction, and obstruction to the rectal outlet were all relieved to a great degree in these patients. 56 % had an overall improvement in symptoms with relief from the varying degrees of extensive symptoms caused by this disease. This again adds to the evidence of the prostatic cancer's radiosensitivity. Evident complications were cystitis and urethritis. We used mainly the linear accelerator and the pelvic rotational techniques, but we did not have any serious complications that necessitated operative intervention. We did get some added depression of the bone marrow, with anaemia especially in those who were also in a poor state of nutrition. I remind you that these were patients with carcinoma of the prostate in stages III and IV and not in the best physical condition. The dosage used (again in a palliative fashion) was 4 − 6,000 rads over a 4 − 6 week period. This was not the high dosage which Dr. *Bagshaw* was using in a potentially curative program.

One of the problems we saw with our patients with prostatic cancer, both those whom we were going to subject to irradiation and those on whom we were going to do a radical prostatectomy, was determination of the extent of the disease and its proper staging. Dr. *Chua* of our department made a study of the bone acid phosphatase in the patients that we were considering for various methods of therapy − not the serum acid phosphatase, but the bone acid phosphatase. His program was to take 10 cc of marrow blood, usually from the iliac bone, and 10 cc of antecubital vein blood, which was immediately placed in the refrigerated centrifuge tube and promptly processed in the laboratory by the Bodanski method. Incidentally, there were 12 patients with benign prostatic hypertrophy, which he also studied, and all 12 of these had normal serum acid phosphatases and normal bone acid phosphatase, as we would expect.

In the prostatic carcinoma group there were 12 patients in clinical stages I and II. All 12 of these had normal serum acid phosphatase, but 4 of them had elevated bone acid phosphatase. In one of these Dr. *Chua* pursued the cancer with a bone biopsy, and found prostatic carcinoma cells. The others had strontium scans, and did not show any evidence of involvement. Incidentally the one that had the positive bone biopsy had a strontium scan which was also negative. A random biopsy picked up the carcinoma. This was indeed unusual. In stage III there were 13 patients. 7 of these were on anti-androgens at the time. 6 had elevated bone acid phosphatase. Of these 6 with elevated bone acid phosphatase, 5 had elevated serum acid phosphatase, but one had a normal serum acid phosphatase. Thus the bone acid phosphatase again seemed more sensitive.

In stage IV of metastatic disease carcinoma were 13 patients. 10 had both bone and serum acid phosphatase elevated; only 2 showed elevated bone acid phosphatase. One had a normal level.

I think Dr. *Chua's* work has given us another tool which we can use quite simply to try to stage the disease more accurately. This may be most helpful to us, not only in evaluating survivals and statistics, but also in selecting forms of therapy.

W. Brosig: I have a question regarding radiotherapy. What happens to the testis? Do you protect the testis when you irradiate the prostate? I remember, one of the first observations that the testis had something to do with cancer of the prostate was made when they irradiated the prostate and did not protect the testis. The results were much better.

W. E. Goodwin: I know, this observation was made by a man named *Munger* in the United States just before *Huggin's* discovery. It was then buried by *Huggin's* work.

M. A. Bagshaw: Dr. *Brosig,* we are very careful not to treat the testis since one of the goals of our therapy is to preserve sexual function. We treat the patient in a standing position – the testes are well below the radiation field. I don't know what would happen if we did otherwise. Of course, spermatogenesis is very radiosensitive, but to destroy the hormone production from the testis takes a much higher dose of radiation.

Dr. Marberger reminded me earlier that radiotherapy is also very useful in the alleviation of painful metastases. This was not the subject of my presentation, but I think it is worthwhile repeating, because many radiotherapists and many urologists do not appreciate that painful bone metastases may be successfully treated by radiotherapy. In fact it is almost as useful as it is in carcinoma of the breast. It does take a slightly higher dose than in breast cancer, and the response is not as rapid, but one can often achieve successful palliation. I have several questions which were handed to me – I'll repeat them. I can hardly answer any of them, but I'll let you know what the questions were.

Does radiosensitivity depend upon the histological grade? I think Dr. Flocks indicated this morning that he thought it did *not,* and I agree with this, but we have not studied it objectively.

Our pathologists have steadfastly refused to grade carcinoma of the prostate, so we have no grade to compare with the radiosensitivity. The one thing that we can say is that even though the tumours seem very well differentiated they are radiosensitive, and will shrink with irradiation.

Does acid phosphatase decrease during therapy? I don't know. We have only studied a few patients and the results were inconclusive.

Did the hormonally-treated patients have a higher stage of disease? I want to emphasise that they did. This probably accounts for the difference in survival rate in our group. I don't think we can attribute the difference in survival to whether or not they had hormones. These were patients who had a longer duration of disease and more advanced disease.

Did patients with elevated serum acid phosphatase have strontium scans? They did not. We were going to initiate a program of doing strontium scans on everyone, but we have not done this yet.

Is the dose at the periphery of the radiation field adequate to treat pericapsular extension? This depends of course on how far the pericapsular extension extends. Our radiation field is either 6X6 cm or 7X7 cm measured at the treatment plane. This is a very small radiation field, and, I think, to achieve these high doses we must keep the field small, but it has to be very precisely aligned. Now with the 6X6 field, we have 4000 rads in a circle that is 12 cm in diameter; and 7500 rads in a circle that is 6 cm in diameter. So, if you consider that most of the periprostatic region is within the 6 cm field, yes, it does receive a high dose. We are still getting 4000 rads at the pelvic margin. If you think for a moment (since we're dealing in solid geometry) a 7X7 cm field treats almost twice the amount of tissue as a 6X6 cm field. If the fields become large, 8X8 or 10X10, then the volume of tissue is appreciably greater, and I would expect more complications.

The Use of Radioactive Isotopes in the Management of Prostatic Cancer

R. H. Flocks

Department of Urology, University of Iowa Hospitals, Iowa City, Iowa, USA

Summary: Curative radiation therapy for cancer of the prostate gland started in 1913. Subsequent experience showed that most of these tumors responded, at least partially, to various modalities of radiation. Two limiting factors were recognized:

1) the complications from radiation of adjacent organs and

2) its ineffectiveness against metastases with death occurring from disseminated tumor. In fact, even today the therapy of metastases is the key in the management of prostatic cancer.

In 1951 interstitial gold radiation (^{198} Au) was instituted by the author as either sole local therapy or as an adjunct to surgery. Metastases have been attacked by external radiation or by intravenous radioactive phosphorus (^{32} P).

Clinical staging divides cases of prostatic cancer into four groups:

Stage 0   =   the operable lesion confined to the prostate gland (2 % of all cases);

Stage I   =   a lesion extending into the seminal vesicles (34 %);

Stage II   =   local extragenital extension (44 %); and

Stage III   =   metastatic lesions (20 %).

Yet further studies point out that up to 45 % of clinical Stage I and Stage II lesions already have metastatic spread via lymphytics and 10 % have spread via the vascular route. Adjunctive use of ^{198} Au in Stage I and II tumors is effective in 50 % of these cases if the lesion is confined locally.

Results of five-year followup in 13 Stage II lesions treated by surgery only showed one patient cured. But, when interstitial ^{198} Au was combined with surgery, 48 of 74 patients were free of disease. Of the 26 failures, only four had local recurrences. Complications of interstitial ^{198} Au are few — mainly delayed wound healing and perineal-urinary fistula. Radiogold as an adjunct to perineal surgery is more effective than ecternal radiation.

Metastatic lesions can be treated with external radiation of 1200–2500 rads in 8 to 18 days. Approximately one-third of prostatic cancers are sensitive to external radiation. Such therapy combined with estrogens is of benefit. Radioactive chromium phosphate and yttrium chloride are not as effective as ^{198} Au and cause significant marrow depression.

After testosterone priming (100 mg intramuscularly every day for five days) ^{32}P can be used for therapy of painful metastases. Minimal marrow depression occurs. The beneficial effects may be due to inhibition of purine synthesis. ^{32}P — polymetaphosphate, two microcuries intravenously, three times weekly, for a total dose of 16 microcuries, is now available for treatment of bone metastases. Combined with estrogen therapy, the effects are synergistic. Side effects are mainly transient leukopenia, nausea, fever and petechiea.

Manuscript received: 14 November 1969

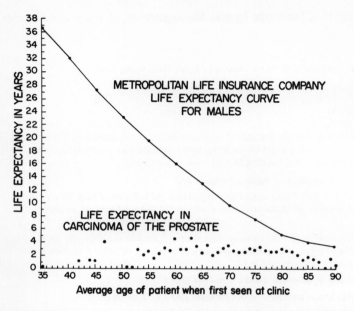

Fig. 1. Life expectancy as compared to normal in 1,249 patients with prostatic cancer followed five years or more and treated by conservative means, including endocrine therapy.

There is a good deal of evidence that many prostatic cancers are radiosensitive to a significant degree. The original works of *Pasteau* and *DeGrais* [1], *Young* [2], *Deming* [3] and *Barringer* [4], at times demonstrated a very striking reduction in the mass of the tumor and they occasionally showed what seemed to be a cure. Similar results were obtained later with radon seeds. More recently, the author's [5–9] results with the interstitial use of [198]Au showed conclusively that many of these tumors were radiosensitive if adequate radiation dosage was utilized. Improved techniques of external irradiation, utilizing either megavoltage or cobalt sources, were described by *George* [10], *Bagshaw* [11], and the author [9]. These have shown very significant changes in the prostatic cancers in approximately 50 % of the patients. No relationship, however, could be demonstrated as far as the grade of the tumor or other histological characteristics were concerned. Tumors of the same grade and also of the same histological appearance, showed different responses to eqivalent doses of irradiation. Survial was related primarily to the stage of the tumor, to the sensitivity of the lesion, and to the magnitude of the radiation dose which could be applied without significant damage to the surrounding structures and the patient as a whole. Fig. 1–3.

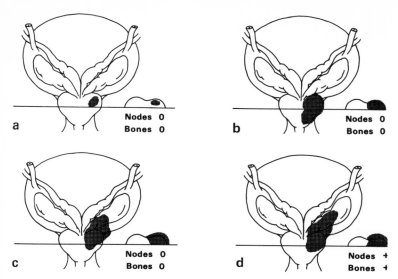

Fig. 2. Staging of prostatic cancer.

a) Lesion completely limited to prostate.

b) Lesion involving most of prostate with possibility of microscopic extension beyond prostate in plane of cleavage of radical prostatectomy.

c) Lesion locally extended beyond prostate to regions of base of bladder and seminal vesicles.

d) Lesion clinically disseminated to lymph nodes and to bones.

It is of interest that extensive clinical and pathological studies have shown that lesions staged a and b show a 10 % incidence of subclinical dissemination and lesions staged c show a 50-75 % incidence of dissemination. These considerations are extremely important when considering survival following only local therapy by any method.

	4500 R or Less	5500 R or More
Marked regression	5	15
Partial regression	7	4
No regression	3	2

Thus 54% of these cancers are quite radiosensitive and this was recognized at the 4500 R point. It is to be emphasized, however, that many of these had residual cancer which became activated at various times after the original treatment - sometimes in a matter of years.

Fig. 3. External radiotherapy to the prostatic area in extracapsular prostatic cancer.

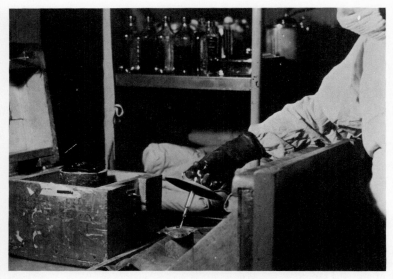

Fig. 4. The radiologist is filling the syringe with the radioactive solution. Not more than 2 cc total volume is utilized. This must contain 40-50 mc of activity per cc.

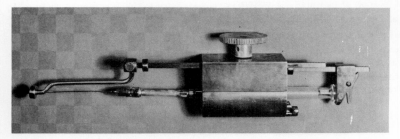

.**Fig. 5.** The lead covered pressure syringe utilized for injection of the radioactive material.

Since 1951, the author has utilized interstitial irradiation with ^{198} Au to destroy or to aid in the destruction of the local lesion in over 1200 patients in several different ways:

(1)   in small operable or large inoperable lesions for the destruction of the entire lesion alone, or in combination with electrosurgical destruction of the main mass of the lesion, and

(2)   as an adjuvant to radical prostatoseminal versiculectomy for inoperable lesions of moderate to large size.

The techniques involved are illustrated in Fig. 4—10 inclusive.

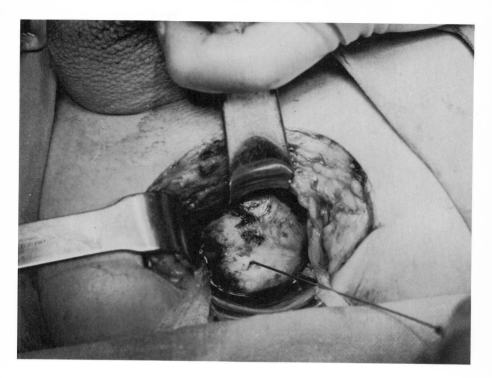

Fig. 6. The prostate exposed perineally and being injected.

The results with regard to the destruction of the local lesion are striking, Fig. 11—14 inclusive.

The results as an adjuvant to radical surgical excision are also striking, Fig. 15—17 inclusive.

As far as changes in the survival figures are concerned, the improvement as compared to a similar group treated palliatively is approximately 30 %. The significance of these figures is hard to estimate because of the high and varying occurrence of metastasis already present at the time of the institution of local therapy. There is no question, however, that this technique will produce complete destruction of the lesion in small operable lesions and in modest to even large sized inoperable lesions with very low morbidity and mortality, and with fewer complications than with radical prostatectomy — no incontinence, no rectal difficulties, and an extremely

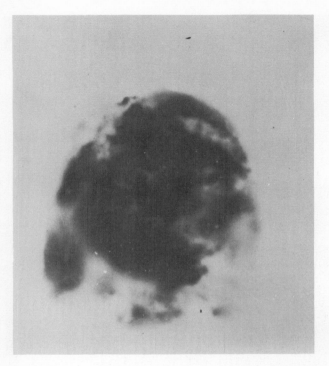

Fig. 7. Radioautograph of prostate after injection of 2 cc of 198 Au solution containing 6 mc of 198 Au. Note character of distribution — about 90 % of the activity remained in the injected area.

low incidence of stricture or other complications. Healing time of the wound is greater than after simple radical prostatectomy and perineal fistula sometimes lasted for several months. The wounds, however, all healed ultimately.

Interstitial irradiation with radioactive gold can be utilized in recurrences after 6500 r delivered externally or after radical prostatectomy. The injection can be performed either transperineally, transrectally, or after perineal exposure of the gland, Fig. 18. A local dosage of 7500 to 15,000 r can thus be introduced into the area in addition to what has been delivered before.

Thus interstitial local treatment with [198] Au is of great significance in the management of the local lesion of prostatic cancer. Because of its flexibility it can deliver a greater dose of radiation to a desired area without complications. When combined

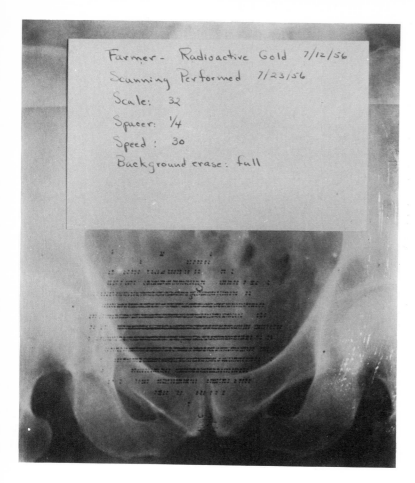

Fig. 8. Scanning of prostatic area 11 days after injection af 198 Au. Note that remaining material in local area is high.

with electrosurgical destruction of the major portion of the lesion, or when combined with prostatoseminal vesiculectomy, it is applicable to a much greater number of patients yielding better results from the point of view of local recurrence and complications than surgery alone or external irradiation alone. It may be safely utilized to give additional therapy to recurrences.

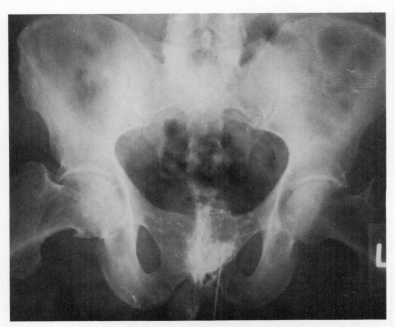

Fig. 9. Monitoring perineal injection by x-ray film of radiopaque material used as a diluent. Note good distribution except about nodule at base of prostate on left side. Such an area can be cauterized with high frequency current and remaining tumor can be destroyed by the combined effect of the 198 Au emissions or more 198 Au solution.

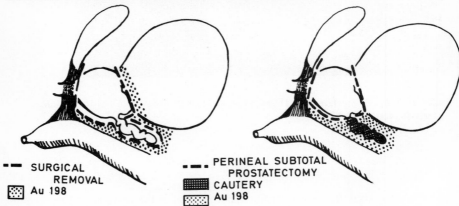

Fig. 10. a) diagram of radical prostatectomy and seminal vesiculectomy with instillation of solution of 198 Au into bed to destroy microscopic extraprostatic extension.

b) diagram of total prostatectomy with destruction of seminal vesicle area by electrocoagulation and then injection of 198 Au solution into bed to destroy extra-prostatic extension.

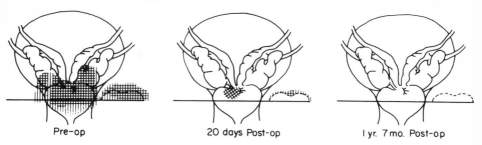

Pre-op   20 days Post-op   I yr. 7 mo. Post-op

Fig. 11. Rectal findings in patient with a large carcinoma which did not respond to estrogen and castration. Injected March, 1951 with 198 Au. Rectal findings 20 days postoperative. Rectal findings 1 year 7 months postoperative. Died 2 years after treatment of cerebrovascular accident – postmortem – no cancer found.

Radioactive isotopes have also been utilized to treat disseminated prostatic cancer. Systemic irradiation with radioactive isotopes for palliation of pain due to disseminated prostatic cancer has been achieved with radioactive phosphorus, ^{32}P, according to *Wildermuth* [12] and associates. In order to enhance the uptake of ^{32}P in tumor-bearing areas, testosterone was given to increase the formation of new bone. An aqueous suspension of 100 mg of testosterone micro-crystals were given daily for five days preceding, during, and for a week following the administration of ^{32}P. Although no conclusions were drawn from the data available to date, *Wildermuth* and associates felt that the extracellular deposition of radioactivity in the area of metastasis was more pertinent in producing the desired effect than intranuclear incorporation. The unexplained minimal hematopoietic inhibition suggests a blocking mechanism according to these authors, who also felt that further investigation of the hormone effect on tumor cells and stroma might demonstrate methods for increasing the ratio of differential absorption. This absorption may also be influenced by dietary and other physiological variations altering the body pool of phosphates. *Wildermuth* stated that the rate of presentation of radioactivity must be balanced against the iso-inhibitory effects on further uptake. This phenomenon was investigated by *Holmes* and *Mee* [13] with external irradiation, as well as chemical agents. Although the dose of X-ray given to the *Jensen* rat sarcoma *in vivo* did actually inhibit desoxyribonucleic acid (DNA) synthesis without at the same time inhibiting synthesis of the protein fractions analyzed, these workers tentatively suggested that it seemed possible that X irradiation produces an inhibition of purine synthesis rather than a direct inhibition of phosphorylation of DNA.

A new ^{32}P labeled Polymetaphosphate has been reported by *Kaplan* [14] and associates to be effective in patients with bone metastasis. It tends to localize in regenerating bones surrounding intra-osseous osteoblastic tumor. Their recommended dosage of 2 millicuries of ^{32}P Metaphosphate intravenously three times

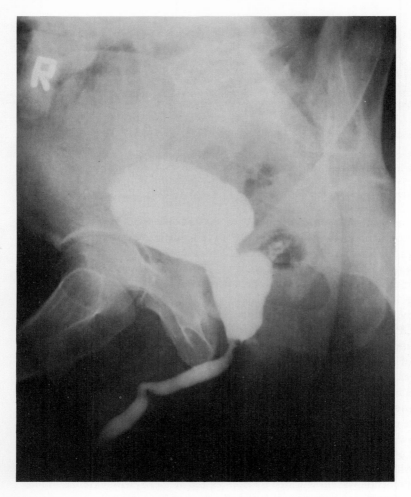

Fig. 12. Cystourethrogram of patient whose prostatic cancer had been treated by combination of electrocoagulation and injection with 85 mc of 198 Au. Note almost complete prostatectomy. Patient is well after five years. He is completely continent.

a week, is given until a dose of 16 millicuries has been given. *Kaplan* reported effective palliation of bone pain, a decrease in alkaline and acid phosphatases, and radiographic regression of lesions. A combination of Polymetaphosphate therapy and estrogen produced a synergistic palliative effect apparently superior to that of either agent alone. Several bedfast patients became ambulatory for the first time

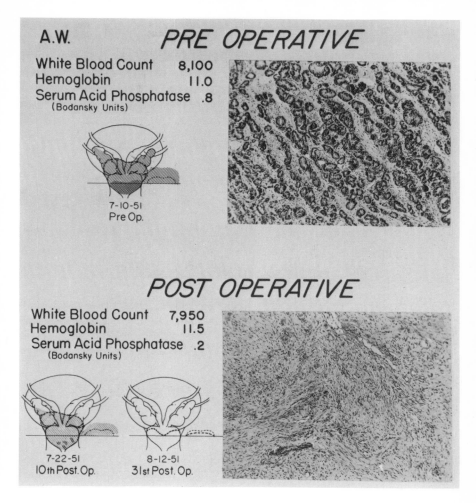

Fig. 13. Rectal findings and histology of patient with prostatic cancer treated by interstitial irradiation with 198 Au in July, 1951. Patient well in September, 1969.

in many months. Transient leukopenia was noted in the patients who experienced clinical benefit. During this post-treatment period, some patients experienced nausea, low-grade fever, and petechiae. The white count did not remain depressed in any instance, even in the presence of progressive anemia. Terminal pneumonia was the apparent cause of death in those patients who died.

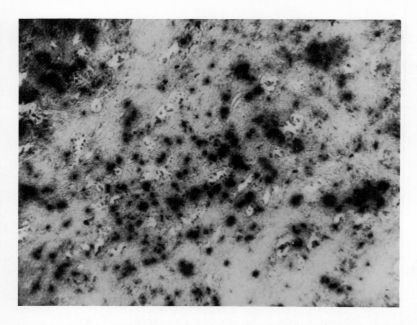

Fig. 14. A microscopic section and superimposed radioautograph of well injected area of prostatic cancer one week after injection. Note quite even distribution of "hot" spots.

	No. of Patients	No. with local Recurrence
Belt [9]	34	8
Scott [9]	29	7
Whitmore and MacKenzie [9]	28	8
Flocks [9]	91*	4

* Solution of ^{198}Au locally instilled used as adjuvant.

Fig. 15. Incidence of local recurrence following surgical removal of prostatic cancer in patients with extraprostatic disease of small extent — patients followed 5 years or more.

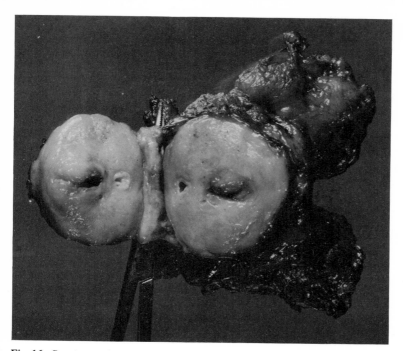

Fig. 16. Prostate and seminal vesicles of patient P. U. Radical retropubic prostatoseminal vesiculectomy and pelvic lymphadenectomy performed in March, 1957. Lymph nodes negative, 198 Au in colloidal solution used as akjuvant. Patient clinically free of cancer September, 1969. Note marked extraprostatic extension of growth. Histologically, growth showed much invasion of perineural lymphatics.

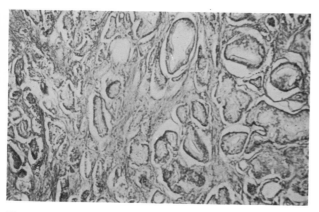

Fig. 17. J. G., age 66, seen July 22, 1954, with prostate as seat of large carcinoma with infiltration around both seminal vesicle areas. Retropubic radical prostatectomy carried out. Pelvic nodes not involved. Bed injected with 50 mc of 198 Au. Note high grade tumor. Alive and well, September, 1969.

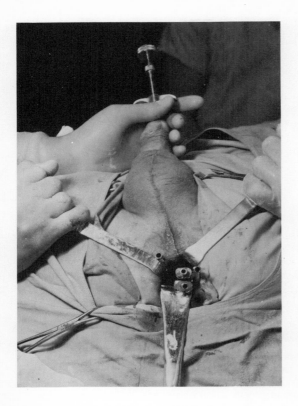

Fig. 18. *Transrectal* injection of 198 Au for recurrence after radical prostatectomy – Needles placed into areas to be injected. These are brought to the operator by a Lowsley tractor.

A series of patients with intractable bone pain and/or rapid deterioration from widely disseminated prostatic cancer nonresponsive to orchiectomy and/or estrogen therapy, were treated with Parathormone, followed by radiophosphorus by *Eddy C. K. Tong* [15] of Brooklyn, New York. The Parathormone was used to create on withdrawal a rebound force that leads to an increased deposition of radiophosphorus in bone and its tumors. The highly energetic beta particles emitted from ^{32}P (1. 7 MeV in peak) can destroy the tumors in bone from within and without. The results of treatment were dramatic. All patients had complete relief of severe pain as well as improvement of the neurological function of lower extremities from epidural metastases. Increase in general strength and appetite, reduction of the elevated serum acid and alkaline phosphatases, recalcification of the eroded pedicles of spine and/or osteolytic lesions elsewhere, and healing of pathological fractures were noted. Depression of bone marrow function was seen in all patients during therapy. However, no serious complication was encountered in any patient and the blood counts usually returned to normal within two months.

These results which are slowly improving are important, not only from a palliative point of view, but also possibly from a curative point of view. They show that the bony metastases from prostatic cancer can be destroyed and it is possible that these might well be destroyed much earlier in their life history and the 5, 10, and 15-year survival of patients increased. The subclinical dissemination frequently present in Stages B and C lesions and high-grade lesions can be destroyed, so that the survival of such patients, after local and disseminated cancer has been thus destroyed, can be significantly enhanced. This might well be carried out by a three-fold attack on suitable cases — pelvic lymphadenectomy, local ablation of the lesion by surgery and irradiation, interstitial or external, and radioisotope therapy intravenously by improved techniques.

In conclusion, prostatic cancer is radiosensitive to a significant but varying degree. Combined surgical and radiation therapy techniques with isotopes offer flexible modalities of therapy. Further clinical studies are needed to utilize these modalities to their utmost, but already very significant improvements in the ablation of the local lesion and much palliation for the disseminated lesions have been achieved.

References

[1] *Pasteau, O.* and *DeGrais:* Radium in treatment of prostatic cancer. J. d'Urologie, Paris, **4**, 3, 341–542, 1913.

[2] *Young, H. H.:* Use of radium in cancer of the prostate and bladder. JAMA, **68**, 1174, 1917.

[3] *Demining, C. L.:* Carcinoma of the prostate and seminal vesicles treated with radium. S. G. & O., **34**, 99, 1922.

[4] *Barringer, B. S.:* Prostatic carcinoma. J. Urol., **33**, 616, 1935.

[5] *Flocks, R. H., Kerr, H. D., Elkins, H. B.* and *Culp, D.:* Treatment of carcinoma of the prostate by interstitial radiation with radioactive gold (^{198}Au): A preliminary report. J. Urol., **68**, 510–522, 1952.

[6] *Flocks, R. H., Kerr, H. D., Elkins, H. B.* and *Culp, D. A.:* The treatment of carcinoma of the prostate by interstitial radiation with radioactive gold (^{198}Au): A follow-up report. J. Urol., **71**, 628–633, 1959.

[7] *Flocks, R. H., Culp, D. A.* and *Elkins, H. B.:* Present status of radioactive gold in manage-
     ment of prostatic cancer. J. Urol., **81**, 178–184, 1959.

[8] *Flocks, R. H.:* Combination therapy for localized prostatic cancer. J. Urol., **89**,
     889–894, 1963.

[9] *Flocks, R. H.:* Interstitial irradiation therapy with a solution of [198]Au as part of com-
     bination therapy for prostatic carcinoma. J. Nuclear Med., **5**, 691–705, 1964.

[10] *George, F. W., Carlton, C. E., Dykhutzen, R. F.* and *Dillon, J. R.:* Cobalt-60 telecurie-
     therapy in the definitive treatment of carcinoma of the prostate: A. preliminary report.
     The Journal of Urology, **93**, 102–109, January 1965.

[11] *Bagshaw, M. A., Kaplan, H. S.* and *Sagerman, R. H.:* Linear accelerator supervoltage
     radiotherapy VII, Cancer of the prostate. Rad. **85**, 121–9, 1965.

[12] *Wildermuth, O., Parker, D., Archambeau, J. O.* and *Chahbazion, C.:* Management of
     diffuse metastases from carcinoma of the prostate. JAMA, **172**, 1607–11, 1960.

[13] *Holmes, B. E.* and *Mee, L. K.:* The incorporation of Methionine ^{35}S into the proteins
     of Jensen rat sarcoma cells after the irradiation of the tumor. Brit. J. Radiology **25**,
     273, 1952.

[14] *Kaplan, E., Fels, I. G., Kotlowski, B. T., Greco, J.* and *Walsh, W. S.:* Therapy of carci-
     noma of the prostate metastatic to bone with ^{32}P labeled condensed phosphate.
     J. Nucl. Med., **1**, 1, 1960.

[15] *Tong, Eddy E. K.:* Parathormone and ^{32}P therapy in prostatic cancer with bone metasta-
     ses. J. Nuc. Med., **10**, 376, 1969.

Discussion

R. H. Flocks: I did not say anything about complications. The complications are, for all practical purposes, nil. In the last 500 patients we have had *one* patient in whom one ureter was
irradiated because the injection went higher than we thought, associated with extension of
the lesion in that area, and this necessitated a reimplantation of the ureter. The wounds however do close much more slowly, so that a wound might very well take several weeks to repair
where previously it would not have. This is all as far as local instillation is concerned.

I would like to say a few words about the difference between retropubic and perineal radical
prostatectomy. I have had experience with both and feel in many ways as Dr. *Kaufman* does,
that there are probably indications for each. However, from the point of view of dealing with
a patient who has received irradiation (I have done radical (or total) prostatectomies following
4500 and 6000 r given externally, primarily to see what 4500 or 6000 r has done), I would
only do this perineally. The morbidity rises quite rapidly when it is done abdominally. My own
preference is the perineal approach, because I can secure a complete visualisation of the prostate, and make a decision whether supplementary therapy with radioactive isotopes is needed
when dealing with a possibly operable case. There is a disadvantage as regards the regional
lymph nodes. We simply do a regional lymph node exploration, as a secondary operation, after
the patient has completely healed and is up and around, after 2 or 3 months, when he's completely recovered from the original operation. Done in this way, the abdominal operative procedure carries a very low morbidity and no mortality, because there is no possibility of urine
contamination. If at that time positive nodes are found in small numbers, a pelvic lymphadenectomy is carried out. If they are found very extensively above the bifurcation of the aorta,
we consider using external irradiation on these nodes.

Irradiation of the Hypophysis for advanced Cancer of the Prostate with Metastases

J. D. Fergusson

Institute of Urology, University of London, England

Rationale: The pituitary gland produces gonadotropins, A. C. T. H., and other hormones thought to be capable of influencing the activity of prostatic cancer. Ablation or destruction of the hypophysis should therefore prevent the secretion of these substances and lead to retardation of the disease. In advanced cases with metastases it is felt that surgical hypophysectomy carries too high an operative risk (10−15 %) for what it is likely to achieve. "Irradiation" hypophysectomy on the other hand is a relatively safe alternative, capable of promoting substantial necrosis of the gland and often producing dramatic symptomatic relief. It has now been used in nearly 100 cases, the first 74 of which (1956−66) provide the substance of this review.

1. Technique

The transnasal inoculation of radioactive material into the pituitary was first developed in the early 1950's for advanced cancer of the breast. At that time small gold seeds were used carrying the isotope ^{198}Au. This substance, a powerful γ-ray emitter with considerable tissue penetration had to be deposited with extreme precision to avoid radiation damage to surrounding structures, notably the optic, oculomotor and trochlear nerves. Accuracy of implantation was assisted by repeated X-ray examination in two planes during the advancement of the introducing needle.

This somewhat time-consuming procedure was later modified by the use of a freehand method of introduction, checked by X-ray screening at intervals in the lateral and antero-posterior planes.

This technique was first adopted for advanced prostatic cancer at St. Paul's Hospital London (Institute of Urology) in the autumn of 1955 and gold seeds were used in the first eight cases. By this time, however, reports were becoming available of several patients who had been similarly treated elsewhere for cancer of the breast and who had developed partial blindness. (Only one of the Institute's cases developed a unilateral field defect).

Manuscript received: 14 November 1969

This led to a search for an alternative source capable of inducing local necrosis yet with more limited tissue-penetration. These desiderata were fulfilled by the isotope ^{90}Y, a pure β ray emitter which could be so prepared as to limit its tissue necrosing effect to a radius of 3—5 mm. This material was used in the ensuing 66 cases in the series.

At the same time the advent of the X-ray Image Intensifier afforded an easier and safer means of screening the alignment of the introducing needle and, when linked with a television monitor, enabled the operator himself to guide its direction. This technique embodying the use of two Image Intensifiers (arranged in the lateral and antero-posterior planes) has now become routine.

The approach to the pituitary fossa may be either transnasal or transethmoidal (via a puncture just medial to the inner canthus). The introducing needle is directed under television-screen control and tapped onwards when necessary with a light hammer until its trocar point penetrates the anterior wall of the sella turcica. The trocar is then removed, leaving the end of the needle abutting on the pituitary gland. A cartridge enclosing the radio-active source is then loaded into the breech of the needle and the pellet propelled into the substance of the gland with a blunt-ended stillette.

To ensure maximum destruction, three pellets of ^{90}Y (each of 3—4 millicuries) are customarily used. These should be distributed (individually) by means of three punctures so as to lie, one in the midline and the other two on each side, in the substance of the gland. It is important that they should not be implanted too high so as to cause damage to the diaphragma sellae and hence leakage of cerebrospinal fluid. Likewise they should not be placed too far back where they may irradiate the pituitary stalk and hypothalamus and induce diabetes insipidus.

It is remarkable how, with a little experience, a suitable distribution can easily be obtained, usually within the space of a few minutes. A short period of general anaesthesia is, of course, obligatory but apart from fitness for this there are few other contra-indications to the use of the technique.

2. Results

In reviewing the results it is important to stress that all the 74 patients were in an advanced and, indeed, penultimate state of the disease. All had previously received estrogens in high dosage (over periods ranging from 3 months to 7 years) and 20 had also been subjected to orchidectomy. With the exception of 2 all had widespread bone metastases and 3 were, in addition, paraplegic. The prime indication for further treatment in these cases was intractable metastatic pain. In the two remaining cases, both of which did badly, the deciding factors were rapid clinical deterioration with recurrent urinary obstruction.

In assessing the response reliance has had to be placed mainly on subjective evidence and on the period of survival. In favourable cases the first indication is an immediate relief of metastatic pain which is frequently dramatic. Within two or three days, unless substitution therapy is commenced, signs of endocrine deficiency begin to obtrude in the form of hypotension and hypoglycemia, with inanition, nausea and coldness of the extremities. These features are combatted by the institution of replacement therapy with cortisone starting on the second postoperative day.

It is perhaps unfortunate that such substitution therapy interferes with hormonal assays both in the blood and urine and prevents accurate assessment of the degree of pituitary hypofunction. Similarly, studies of iodine uptake by the thyroid during the postoperative period have given equivocal results. Nevertheless in responsive cases there can be little doubt about the symptomatic benefit.

3. Symptomatic response

This has been recorded in three grades, namely: —

(1) Good   implying complete relief from metastatic pain continuing over a substantial period of months or years.

(2) Intermediate   typified by significant relief followed by ultimate relapse.

(3) Poor   denoting no appreciable benefit.

Approximately two-fifths of the cases (31 patients) qualified for the first category. Among these were two of the three paraplegic patients, and both were restored to ambulation having previously been bedridden. Survival in this group ranged from 4 months to $3\frac{1}{2}$ years with an average of just over one year.

20 patients fell into the intermediate category showing significant relief for a shorter period, with survival varying between one and seven months.

23 patients (about $\frac{1}{3}$ of the series) derived no appreciable benefit and included two cases in which death occurred within a few days of implantation. The average survival in this category was only 3 weeks.

4. Age

Analysis by age shows little of importance apart from emphasizing that many of the patients were decidedly elderly. This is to some extent reflected in the greater number of poor results obtained in the highest age group (over 70 years) in which death might well be expected from intercurrent disease.

5. Complications

Despite the fact that the intervention is a minor one and well tolerated by the frailest of patients, it would be idle to suggest that there is no risk of complications.

These in the main stem from misplacement of the radioactive seeds and tend to diminish with increasing experience.

Visual field defects (which may be delayed) and oculomotor disturbances occurred only twice in the series both in early cases when γ-emitting gold seeds were used.

Transient polyuria has been a common feature in cases when the radio-active source has been lodged too far posteriorly. Spontaneous recovery has been the rule, aided on occasions by the temporary use of pituitary snuff or injections of pitressin tannate.

Leakage of cerebrospinal fluid of varying degree occurred in 20 patients, mainly among the earlier cases in which implantation was less accurate. The roof of the sella is often concave (like a saucer) and it is important to avoid placing the seeds too high and risking radionecrosis. In most instances the leakage was self-terminating but in one case the fistula had to be closed by formal trans-ethmoid hypophysectomy.

Infective complications were rare, possibly mainly on account of the local sterilizing effect of the radio-active source. Nevertheless antibiotic cover was prescribed as a routine to cover the immediate postoperative period. There were two instances of transient meningism, and one case probably died of meningitis.

This catalogue of possible complications should not be construed as unduly forbidding since, for the most part, the ill effects have been transient. When equated with the symptomatic benefit and prolonged survival which may well accrue there can be little doubt that such hazards are reasonably acceptable. It should be emphasized, however, that "irradiation" hypophysectomy remains the ultimate expedient in endocrine therapy and should be restricted solely to cases failing to respond to simpler measures.

Discussion

J. D. Fergusson: I have had one question: How do you explain the dramatic relief of pain in such a short period after the operation, because after a formal surgical hypophysectomy the pain is very often not relieved for a longer period? I cannot explain this, except that I do not believe that it is due to concussion, as the patients are usually awake about 1/2 hour after the implantation and reading their evening papers.

My contribution was a factual one and there is not very much that I can add, except to say that we have now done 104 cases, and the same pattern of symptomatic relief emerges. One cannot predict in advance which cases are going to respond and which are not, but there is a slight difference in those patients who have previously been orchiectomised. They do not responds quite as well as patients who still have their testes. One would expect this, since the effect is probably mediated, partly through the testis.

Cytotoxic Agents in the Treatment of Prostatic Carcinoma

G. Jönsson

Urological Clinic, University Hospital, Lund, Sweden

Summary: Reports on the treatment of advanced prostatic carcinoma with substances that have been proved to have a cytotoxic effect are few and opinions differ on the evaluation of the results obtained. There is some evidence that prostatic carcinoma is sensitive to alkylating agents.

During the last two years, we at the Urological Clinic in Lund, Sweden, have been running a pilot trial with *Estracyt*. This preparation is an estradiol in phosphate form which is by a carbamate link fixed to nor-nitrogen-mustard gas. The preparation is given intravenously. The treated series consisted of 65 patients. All the patients had metastases. The acid phosphatases were increased in 42 patients. 3–4 g have been given over 10–20 days before the response to the therapy could be assessed. Some patients have received 50 g of *Estracyt*. A marked improvement was recorded in 38 cases. A striking feature was the disappearance of bone pain. In 9 patients, the metastases have been reduced or resolved. The value of acid phosphatases generally dropped to normal values when the patient improved. Pathological and cytological investigation of the prostate before and during the treatment sometimes showed marked regressive changes. Slight leucopenia and thrombopenia have been recorded in 5 patients. The most common side effect is the thrombophlebitis at the site of injection.

The therapeutic methods available for treatment of cancer fall into four groups; namely surgery, radiation, chemotherapy and hormone therapy. Each of these methods may be used by itself or combined with one or more of the others. So far, hormone therapy and chemotherapy are used mainly as supplementary measures to the first two methods (Fig. 1).

Chemotherapy or treatment with cytostatic and cytotoxic substances are relatively new methods, but have already produced very promising results and there is reason to believe that they might one day become the methods of choice.

It might not be out of place first to give a brief recapitulation of some of the milestones in the development of our treatment of carcinoma (Fig. 2).

Manuscript received: 14 November 1969

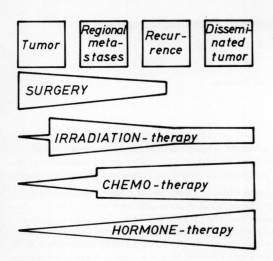

Fig. 1
Methods available for treatment of carcinoma.

We see that the first two observations date far back into time and were made at extirpation of the gonads. From 1939 several clinically valuable discoveries have been made. We are all well acquainted with *Huggins'* observations as well as with the significance of the nitrogen mustard in the treatment of certain tumours.

Also the history of anticancer drugs has some milestones (Fig. 3).

Thus, in the early 1940s, estrogens were used in the treatment of metastatic prostatic cancer, and both sex hormones were given to patients with advanced breast cancer. After the last World War, the alkylating agents were presented (trimethylenemelamine (TEM), chlorambucil, thio-Tepa, busulphan and cyclophosphamide).

In rapid succession, the folic acid antagonists, the adrenal steroids, actinomycin D, and 6-mercaptopurine became available. Since 1954, the new major drugs of practical value include 5-fluorouracil, the progestational hormones and the vinca alkaloids (vinblastine and vincristine). Compounds of less or unproved value are mitomycin C, methylhydrazin and cytosine.

The commonest anti-cancer drugs are usually divided into five groups according to their mode of action and origin (Fig. 4).

Time will not allow a detailed description of the mode of action of these drugs.

Treatment of advanced carcinoma of the prostate is a large field offering many obstinate problems. Though we can now offer our patients good palliation with conventional operative, hormone and general supplementary therapy, sooner or later the disease will progress. In other words we can delay, but not prevent the fatal progression of the disease.

Year	Event or Observation
1837	Orchiectomy - Regression of prostate (Civiale)
1896	Ovariectomy - Regression of mammary carcinoma (Beatson)
1898	Dimethyleneimine - Necrosis of renal papillae (Ehrlich)
1936	Estrogen - Stimulation of mouse mammary carcinoma (Lacassagne)
1939	Estrogen and castration - Regression of prostatic secretion (Huggins et al.)
1942	Nitrogen mustard - Regression of lymphosarcoma (Gilman & Philips)
1942	Purine analogs - Blocking of nucleic acid synthesis (Hitchings et al.)
1943	Mustard gas - Depression of leukocyte formation (Alexander)
1946	Urethan - Tumor inhibition (Haddow & Sexton)
1948	Aminopterin - Remission in leukemia (Farber et al.)
1950	Actinomycin - Antitumor activity (Stock)
1953	6-mercaptopurine - Remission in myel. leuk. (Burchenal et al.)

Fig. 2. Historical highlights.

With the advent of chemotherapy, it was hoped that new and effective methods of treatment of carcinoma would become available. Various trials with new cytotoxic agents have been reported, but such agents have been tried less often in the treatment of prostatic carcinoma, and the results obtained have been less favourable.

Hormone therapy with estrogens is referred to in the literature as cytotoxic chemotherapy, but since the effect of estrogens by inhibition of gonadotropin has already been discussed at this meeting, I will not dwell longer on this point.

Several of the estrogens used are, however, believed to have a direct effect on the cancer cell, though convincing evidence of such an effect is still missing. Even *Huggins* suggested the possibility of such a direct cytotoxic effect because several series on record appear to show that orchiectomy + Stilbestrol produced a better effect than orchiectomy alone.

1935

  Estrogens, androgens; Nitrogen mustard

1945 Antifolics; Adrenal steroids

1950

  Mercaptopurine: Chlorambucil

  Thio-TEPA; Busulfan; Actinomycin D

1955

  Fluorouracil; Cyklophosphamide

  Progestins

1960 Vinblastine; Vincristine

  Metylhydrazine; Cytosine

1965

Fig. 3. Historical development of anti-cancer drugs.

Alkylating agents: Nitrogen mustards
        thio-TEPA; Chlorambucil
Busulfan; Melphalan; Cyklophosphamide

Antimetabolites: Metrotrexate
5-Fluorouracil; 6-Mercaptopurine

Steroid hormones: Androgens; Estrogens
Adrenal cortical steroids; Progestational agents

Antibiotics: Actinomycin D

Plant alkoloids: Vinblastine; Vincristine

Fig. 4. Classes of anti-cancer drugs.

Today, I will discuss especially two preparations, namely diethyl-dioxystilbenedi-phosphate and polyestradiolphosphate. The former preparation is known under the name of *Honvan*. It is a water-insoluble phosphorylated stilbene and was first employed clinically by *Druckrey* and *Raabe* [3] and credited with specific effects on the prostatic cancer cells. They and other clinicians assumed that it would penetrate into the normal and neoplastic epithelial cell and become dephosphorylated by their acid phosphatases. This would then result in a precipitation of the stilbene compound in the prostatic cell. Those who used this preparation and published their results do not

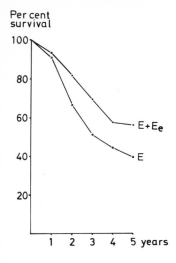

Fig. 5

Cancer prostatae – Survival rate after Estradurin and Estradurin + etinyl-estradiol.

appear to have obtained a better effect than with other estrogens. Investigations by, among others, *Rothauge* et al. [16] and *Fergusson* [5] however, seem to have shown that the preparation exerts its effect mainly via inhibition of pituitary gonadotropin.

Polyestradiol phosphate is a polymerization product of phosphorylated estradiol. This preparation was introduced after clinical trials at our clinic. The preparation is given i.m. once a month in a dose of 80–160 mg. Steroid metabolic studies showed that with these doses only a relatively mild inhibition of gonadotropin was obtained. But this inhibition could be strengthened by increasing the doses. Estradurin is a strong enzyme inhibitor. Since the results were good and better than those obtained with gonadotropin inhibiting substances, and since patients, who from the very beginning did not respond to ordinary estrogen therapy or after treatment with stilbestrol failed to do so, reacted favourably to polyestradiol, it was assumed that the effect of the preparation was exerted on the cancer cells, possibly by its antienzymatic effect.

Combined treatment with a strong gonadotropin inhibitor, etinyl-estradiol, and a strong enzyme inhibitor, Estradurin, was found to give a five year survival rate of 60 %, the corresponding figure for Estradurin alone in a comparative series being only 39 % (Fig. 5).

In summary, one may say that accumulated evidence indicates an indirect action of estrogens on prostatic cancer in man by way of the inhibition of pituitary gonado-tropins. A direct effect of estrogens upon prostatic cancer has not been proved, but has been considered as a result of tissue culture and *in vitro* metabolic studies [8, 10, 12, 13].

Reports on the treatment of advanced prostatic carcinoma with substances that have been proved to have a cytotoxic effect are few and opinions differ on the evaluation of the results obtained.

There is some evidence that prostatic carcinoma is sensitive to alkylating agents [6]. *Flocks* and co-workers recently reported 14 cases treated with mustard gas. In two of these cases, where the substance was given intra-aortally and the prostate was perfused, histological examinations showed severe destruction of the canceromatous tissue. The other 12 cases with disseminated lesions reported that they felt better after such treatment. Pain disappeared and remission occurred in 50 % of the cases. The relief was, however, of short duration. In order to achieve the best possible effect on carcinoma and the least possible injury to normal cells, mustard gas was given at 5 week intervals. Such intervals are not long enough for the carcinoma to be able to progress, but they are long enough for the bone marrow to replace itself and return to normal. This is because „the doubling time" of prostatic carcinoma is markedly longer than that of the bone marrow.

Another alkylating substance, thio-TEPA, has also been tried in the treatment of prostatic carcinoma. Thus, *Weyrauch* and *Nesbet* [18] reported that 4 cases of prostatic carcinoma were treated with local injections intermittently, at monthly intervals. The patients reported that they felt better, and objective signs of regression of the growth were noted and histological examination showed signs of destruction of the cancer epithelium.

Cyclophosphamide (Endoxan, Cytoxan), which also belongs to the alkylating substances has also been tried in the treatment of prostatic carcinoma. *Fox* [7] thus reported that out of 20 patients with urological carcinoma, 4 had carcinoma of the prostate. Of these, 1 showed objective signs of regression, 2 reported that they felt better, and one did not respond at all. Similar observations have been reported by *Rockstroh* et al. [15], *Hammer* and *Enderlein* [9] and *Shnider* et al. [17].

In 1967, *Arduino* and *Mellinger* [2] reported their experience in the treatment of 16 patients with advanced carcinoma of the prostate. The patients were treated with Busulfan, which is also an alkylating substance. 2 mg were given twice a day. The authors concluded that Busulfan is of little or no value in the treatment of prostatic carcinoma and that the toxic myelosuppression was very strong.

In 1965, *Falkson* and *Falkson* [4] reported the results of treatment of 24 patients with advanced carcinoma. Five of these had prostatic carcinoma. All the patients received Serincarbamate ester (Camosin). One of these showed objective signs of improvement: the acid phosphatases became normal and the osteolytic metastases became sclerotic. After 7 months, an exacerbation occurred. The other four experienced a short improvement of bone pain, but no objective signs of improvement. Camosin often produced side effects in the form of nausea, vomiting, diarrhoea, leucopenia and anaemia.

In the investigations by *Flocks*, which I mentioned just now, also 5-Fluorouracil was used combined with nitrogen mustard. It is probably impossible to decide which of these substances produced the improvement reported.

Arduino [1] also reported that he tried Cytoxan (cyclophosphamide) on 7 patients with prostatic carcinoma. In none of these patients did it produce any demonstrable effect on the tumour, the symptoms or the clinical course.

Of the antibiotics, Actinomycin D appears hardly to have been used, but *Mackenzie, Duruman* and *Whitmore* [14] tried Mitramycin in 6 patients, and *Kofman* and *Eisenstein* [11] in 7 with prostatic cancer. The latter reported subjective improvement in all, regression of metastases in two, and reduction of serum acid phosphatase in three.

Mackenzie and co-workers [14] could report only reduction of pain in three patients. There was no regression of the tumour and no reduction of serum acid phosphatase. The toxic side-effects were severe.

During the last two years we at my clinic have been running a pilot trial with Estracyt. The preparation is an estradiol in phosphate form, which by a carbamate link is fixed to nor-nitrogen-mustard gas. By enzymatic splitting by the carbamidase, the nor-nitrogen-mustard gas is released from the estradiol phosphate. The preparation is given intravenously (Fig. 6).

Estracyt is biologically inactive until it is split. It is yet unknown exactly where or to which extent the injected substance is decomposed.

The treated series consisted of 67 patients, including 65 with advanced prostatic carcinoma, one with bladder carcinoma and one with colonic carcinoma. In 38 of the 65 cases of prostatic carcinoma, the grade of differentiation is reported and it appears that 21 had a poorly differentiated, 13 a fairly well differentiated, and 4 a highly differentiated tumour (Fig. 7).

Skeletal metastases were present in 54 patients, in most cases they were very widespread. Soft tissue metastases have been observed in 18 patients. These have been mainly palpable resistances near the bladder or overgrowth towards the rectum and peritoneum as well as lymph node metastases. Pulmonary metastases have been observed in 6 patients, 15 patients showed a multiple localization of these three types (Fig. 8).

The therapeutic period has varied considerably according to the reaction of the patients. 3—4 have been given over 10—20 days before the response to the therapy could be assessed.

However, in certain cases a good response was noted already after 1—2 g. Some patients have received 50 g Estracyt. If no effect was observed after 3 g, treatment was discontinued. When improvement was observed, the injections were continued until the patient had been rendered as symptom free as possible.

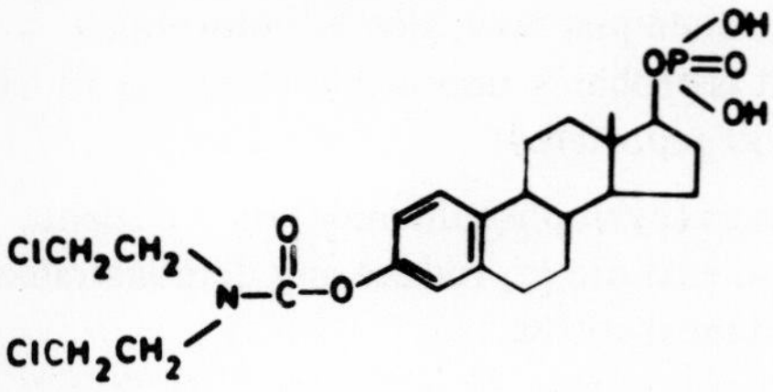

Fig. 6. ESTRACYT.

Poorly	Intermediate	Highly	Unknown
21	13	4	27

Skeletal	Soft tissue	Pulm.
54	18	6

Fig. 7. Differentiation (65).   **Fig. 8.** Metastases (65).

The effect of this therapy is not yet entirely clarified. However, a marked improvement was recorded in 28 cases, and a significant improvement for a shorter or longer period in 12 cases. In 9 cases, the condition has remained unchanged, while no response was observed in 18 cases, who continued to deteriorate. A striking feature was the disappearance of bone pain. Many patients were able to do without their large doses of analgetics, and bedridden patients became mobile and active. Troublesome dysuria had also disappeared.

In 9 patients, the metastases have been reduced or resolved (2 skeletal-, 4 soft tissue- and 3 pulmonary metastases). The occasionally very high values of acid phosphatase generally dropped to normal values and this drop has most often been associated with a marked improvement (27 patients). When no change in the values of acid phosphatase occurred during the treatment, the patient has usually not responded to this therapy.

A pathological and cytological investigation of the prostate before and during the treatment sometimes showed marked regressive changes which are undoubtedly related to the time of administration of the substance. These changes have been observed in spite of preceding longterm estrogen therapy and have been rather different in character from those produced by estrogen therapy.

The most common side-effect has been the thrombophlebitis which occurred at the site of injection. In most cases, an arterio-veneous shunt was made on the forearm to facilitate the injections.

Slight leucopenia and thrombopenia have been recorded in 5 patients and the therapy has therefore been discontinued for shorter or longer periods, awaiting the normalization of leucocyte and thrombocyte counts. Transitory jaundice was recorded in 2 patients.

It is not possible to say anything definite about these results, but in about 50 % it is possible to achieve considerable alleviation of pain. Objective changes were noted in the metastases, acid phosphatases and the histological picture of the cancer.

The preparation should not replace the conventional therapy, but should be regarded as a very useful adjuvant, where other forms of therapy fail.

Summing up, the treatment of advanced prostatic carcinoma still offers several obstinate problems. Treatment with cytostatics has so far not been so very promising. Nevertheless, there is reason to hope that new advances in cytotoxics will sooner or later appear and improve the effect of such agents.

References

[1] *Arduino, L. J.:* Chemotherapy in Urologic Cancer, Surg. Clin. of N. Amer., **45**, 1351 (1965).

[2] *Arduino, L. J. & Mellinger, G. T.:* Clinical Trial of Busulfan (NSC–750) in Advanced Carcinoma of Prostate. Cancer Chemotherapy Rep., **51**, No. 5, Sept., 295 (1967).

[3] *Druckrey, H. & Raabe, S.:* Organspezifische Chemotherapie des Krebses (Prostatacarcinom). Klin. Wschr. 30, 882 (1952).

[4] *Falkson, G. & Falkson, H. C.:* DL-Serine Bis (2-Chloropropyl) Carbamate Ester (CB–3210; NSC–37023) for Treatment of Cancer Patients – Preliminary Results. Cancer Chemotherapy Rep. No. 49, Dec 31 (1965).

[5] *Fergusson, J. D.:* Tracer Experiments showing the Distribution and Fate of Injected Phosphorylated Estrogens in Cancer of the Prostate. Brit. J. Urol. 33, 442 (1961).

[5] *Flocks, R. H. & Shu-Feng Cheng:* Combination Therapy for Prostatic Carcinoma. J. of Iowa Med. Soc. **58**, No. 2, 125 (1969).

[7] *Fox, M.:* The Effect of Cyklophosphamide on some Urinary Tumours. Brit. J. Urol. 37, 399 (1965).

[8] *Franks, L. M.:* The Effects of Age on the Structure and Response to Estrogens and Testosterone of the Mouse Prostate in Organ Cultures. Brit. J. Cancer 13, 59 (1959).

[9] *Hammer, O. & Enderlein, G.:* Med. Welt 37, 1750 (1960).

[10] *Knobil, E.:* The Relation of some Steroid Hormones to Beta-Glucuronidase Activity. Endocrinology **50**, 16 (1952).

[11] *Kofman, S. & Eisenstein, R.:* Mitramycin in the Treatment of Disseminated Cancer. Cancer Chemotherapy Rep., **32**, 77 (1963).

[12] *Lasnitzki, I.:* The Effect of Estrone alone and combined with 20-methylcholanthrene on Mouse Prostate Glands Grown *in vitro*. Cancer Res. **14**, 632 (1954).

[13] *MacDonald, D. F. & Latta, M. J.:* Aerobic Glycolysis of Human Prostatic Adenoma: *in vitro* Inhibition by Estrogen and by Androgen and Estrogen. Endocrinology 59, 153 (1956).

[14] *Mackenzie, A. R., Duruman, N. & Whitmore Jr., W. F.:* Mithramycin in Metastatic Uro-
      genital Cancer. J. of Urology, **98**, 116 (1967).

[15] *Rockstroh, H., Hasselbacher, K. & Barth, F.:* Bruns Beiträge. Klin. Chir. **199**, 355. (1959).

[16] *Rothauge, C. F., Weller, O. & Schuchardt, E.:* Die Wirkung von Diäthyldioxystilbendi-
      phosphat (Honvan®) auf die Keimdrüse und die Gonadotropinausscheidung beim Manne.
      Klin. Wschr. **41**, 90 (1963).

[17] *Shnider, J., Gold, I.:* Cancer Chemotherapy Rep. **8**, 106 (1960).

[18] *Weyrauch, H. M. & Nesbet, J. D.:* Use of Triethylene Thio-Phosphoramide (Thio-Tepa)
      in the Treatment of Advanced Carcinoma of Prostate. J. Urol. **81**, 185 (1959).

Discussion

B. L. R. A. Coolsaet*: **Experiences with 84 cases treated with Honvan** *(stilboestrol diphosphate) 500 mg intravenously per day, during 10 days, in the symptomatic treatment of prostatic carcinoma*

After the convincing publication of *Mellinger*, 1 mg of stilboestrol daily is the indicated treatment, combined or not with total orchidectomy and corticosteroids.

Awaiting further differentiation of the prostatic carcinoma and the determination of its dependence on oestrogens on the basis of histopathologic differentiation and extensive endocrinologic examination, we treated a number of patients with stilboestrol diphosphate (Honvan) intravenously in a dosage of 500 mg daily during 10 days.

Our investigations with Honvan can be divided into two groups: The *first group* refers to the primary treatment of prostatic carcinoma stages III and IV with serious dysuria and/or pains; the *second group* relates to the treatment of patients with prostatic carcinoma stage IV, who have grown resistant to stilboestrol-therapy.

1st Group

This group consists of 42 patients in stage III and IV.

In the cases of stage III, 6 of the patients complained of serious pains, that disappeared after the cure in all 6 cases.

6 Patients had dysuria-complaints with more than 100 ml of residual urine; in 3 of them this volume decreased to normal limits.

33 stage IV – patients were treated, 26 of which had violent pains caused by the metastases, and a bad general condition; 17 (± 65 %) of them were free of complaints after the cure.

Dysuria was present in 12 patients; in 5 of these cases the residual urine was reduced to normal limits after the cure.

* Department of Urology, De Wever-kliniek, Heerlen, The Netherlands.

In 90 % of the cases, the alcaline phosphatase activity was increased at the end of the cure; the acid phosphatase levels were decreased until normal values in 90 % of the cases.

2nd Group

28 Patients with carcinoma of the prostate, stage IV, resistant to therapy with stilboestrol, were treated in the same way; 12 of them were treated two times, one patient had 3 cures of treatment.

At the beginning of the cure with Honvan the patients showed a deterioration of the general condition, complaints of backache with ischiadiformic irradiation and two times there was an invasion of the tumour into the lumen of the rectum.

The reason for treatment was in 12 cases the appearance of dysuria with more than 100 ml of residual urine; in 9 (that is 2/3) of these cases the micturition difficulties disappeared during the cure. In 3 others a transurethral resection was necessary. 29 Patients complained of violent pains, which disappeared in 18 (about 60 %) during the cure.

In contradistinction to what we observed in the first group of patients, the acid phosphatase levels were raised in 90 % after the treatment in this second group, while the alkaline phosphatases in contrary were decreased in 90 % of the cases.

Complications

- The 1st, 5th and 10th day of the cure the electrolytes were measured; no serious alterations could be observed.
- The 5th and 10th day, a complete examination of the coagulation-factors was done; in all cases normal values were found.
- In four cases an increase of bilirubinemia was observed, although no livermetastases could be demonstrated.
- The cure was stopped in two cases because of drug-fever, in two other cases owing to vomitus.
- 6 patients died during the cure, from severe pulmonary embolism.
- 8 cases were treated with a cure according to the same dosage-scheme, although the general condition of these patients was very bad with severe cachexia; they died during the treatment.
- 1 Patient died, on the 3rd day of the cure, from a total consumption-coagulopathy; we did not find similar reports in the literature.
- 1 Patient showed a hyperthermic syndrome; the second day of treatment a condition of subcoma developed, with compulsive upward position of the eyes. EEG and bloodpressure were normal; pulse rate 120 per minute; normal coagulation-status. The biochemical tests did not show abnormalities. There were no signs of sepsis. After some hours a coma-like condition developed with strabismus divergens. Temp. 43°, exitus.

  Conclusion of the postmortem-examination-report: extensive metastases in the liver; centres of demyelinisation in the brain, on the right near the insula.

Discussion

Although our experiences with high dosages of intravenous Honvan in 84 cures of treatment is limited, we can draw some conclusions that may be useful.

Remarkable is the great number of patients that died during the cure, what we did not find earlier mentioned in the literature. It is said, that not much benefit can be expected with patients who are in a bad general condition. Our finding is, that a cure with such high dosages is very dangerous in these patients.

Probably stilboestrol diphosphate exerts a direct toxic effect upon the carcinoma cell. In case of extensive dissemination of metastases one is right to assume that too massive liberation of these toxic products from the destructed tumour-tissue is to be feared in those patients with strongly decreased resisting-power.

The high percentage of increased acid phosphatase levels following the treatment may give evidence for that.

This is the only way in which we can explain the course of the disease in the 2 last patients that we described.

For these reasons we have started a new series on the following scheme:

	morning	afternoon	evening	
1st day	125 mg		125 mg	(Honvan intra-venously)
2nd day	125 mg		125 mg	
3rd day	125 mg	125 mg	125 mg	
4th day	125 mg	125 mg	125 mg	
5th day	250 mg		250 mg	
6th day	500 mg			

and so on, until the acid phosphatase levels are normal.

We treated 23 patients according to this scheme until now and did not see any complication.

We are of opinion that stilboestrol diphosphate is a good product, but it can be dangerous in some cases when treating the severe complicating symptoms occuring in the course of prostatic carcinoma stage IV.

G. Jönsson: I should like to add that the material I presented was not from my own hospital, because I do not have so many cases of advanced prostatic carcinoma. It was from 10 hospitals in southern Sweden. It is collected material. The question for me and for all of us has been: can I do something for the patient with an advanced prostatic carcinoma and severe pain? If a man who was treated for 3 or 4 years with oestrogens comes in with uraemia and obstruction of both ureters, with a big mass in the pelvis, you give him a cytotoxic agent. Two years later he is living and working without pain. So in some cases I think we can gain some benefit from these preparations. I cannot do a hypophysectomy in such a case and I don't think you can.

A. Sigel: Dr. *Flock's* idea of manipulating prostatic cancer by local injections of radioactive gold was the reason why my collaborators and I initiated local cold (*not* gold), therapy with liquid nitrogen. We have constructed a cold pistol, but our experience is only *very* elementary. I wish to stress the term "elementary". Cold therapy by means of trans-urethral techniques is usually not lethal to cancer cells, due to reasons I will not describe now. External open perineal use of liquid nitrogen with certain variations has perhaps a real chance to become one of the good methods for combating prostatic cancer.

W. E. Goodwin: I think, the subject of cryotherapy is very important. Maybe this can be discussed by the panel this afternoon.

F. Schroeder: **Tissue culture studies — preliminary report**

During this conference the importance of growing human prostatic carcinoma cells *in vitro* for experimental purpose has been stressed on several occasions. In spite of great efforts to do so, this has not yet been achieved. Professor *L. Röhl* gave us a brief report on his work in Lund (Sweden) ten years ago (Acta Chir. Scand. 715, suppl. 240 (1959))and pointed out that the hormone dependency of his tissue cultures was always lost after a few generations of growth. Similar observations were made by *J. Lanitzki* in London (J. Natl. Cancer Inst. 65, 339 (1965)) in organ cultures of rat ventral prostate. The most satisfying explanation for this spontaneous loss of the hormone responsive properties of the cells under tissue culture conditions is overgrowth of stromal tissues or other non-hormone dependent cells.

Presently working with the research group we are around Dr. *Gordon Sato* at the University of California at San Diego. This group has been quite successful in growing hormone dependent cells like Leydig cells, adrenal cells, and those of melanomas and pituitary tumors in monolayer tissue cultures. Their techniques appear likely to avoid the problems that prohibited succes in the past. They allow selective growth of hormone dependent cells and eradication of non-hormone dependent cells. The techniques in use will not be described in this preliminary report.

These tissue culture methods have now been applied to three human prostate carcinomas, all were parts of total perineal prostatectomy specimens supplied by the Elmer Belt Urological Group in Los Angeles. The tumor referred to as EBl, a grade III carcinoma is now growing in its fourth week in the manner the following figures (Fig. 1–4) show.

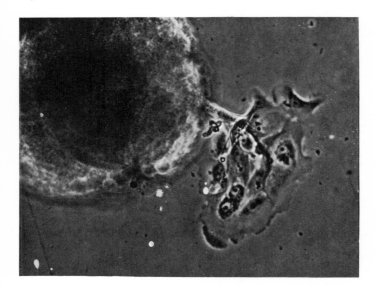

Fig. 1. It can be seen here that a few cells are growing out of a small piece of tumor. The cells are spread out at the bottom of the tissue culture flask and are adherent to it. This photomicrograph is taken through a phase contrast microscope with a magnification of 200. The picture was taken on the fifth day after plating of the tumor.

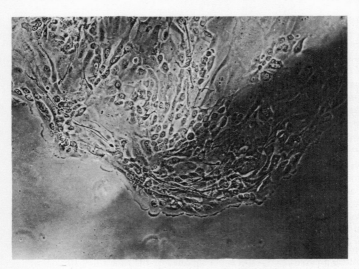

Fig. 2. It is obvious that 2 days later the number of cells has markedly increased. They grow in one layer and details can be recognized in the nuclei and cytoplasm. Dividing cells have frequently been observed.

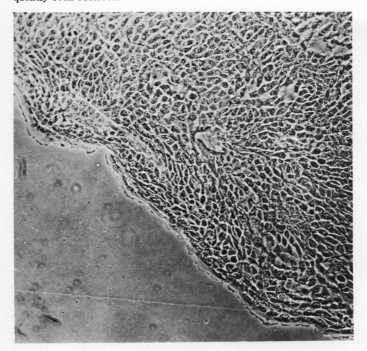

Fig. 3. After several days most of the bottom space in the flask was filled as can be seen. Subculturing was undertaken at this time.

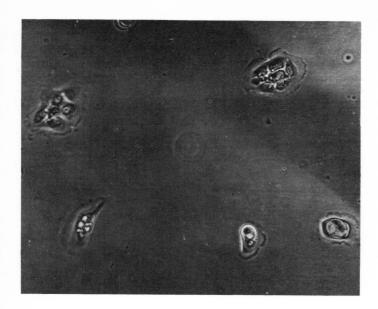

Fig. 4. After trypsinizing the cells to lift them off the plastic material, it is possible by dilution to single out cells like the group shown here.

If the original culture contained several unknown cell types this is one of the methods by which these can be separated from one another and isolated in subculture for further growth. Chance determines which type of cell will be picked up and in which flask only stroma cells, mixed populations or carcinoma will come to grow.

Unfortunately there is no way to recognize cells growing in a culture as cancer cells, fibroblasts or others microscopically. It will be necessary to identify these cells by their specific properties of hormone dependency, production of acid phosphatase, citric acid and other biological characteristics. A first step was taken using *Burstone's (Kaplow, L. S.* and *Burstone, M. W.,* Nature, 200, 690 (1963))* histochemical technique for acid phosphatase determination. Acid phosphatase was demonstrated in the cultured cells just like it was in fresh frozen sections of the original tissue.

The possibility of developing a stabile and reproducible culture model of human prostate cancer for the study of basic problems such as metabolic mechanisms of hormone dependence and resistence as well as the purpose of working out a culture technique simple enough to be used as a hormone sensitivity test for cancer of the prostate are strong stimuli to the attainment of success in our work.

Experiences with Cyproterone Acetate and Related Drugs in the Treatment of Prostatic Disease

W. E. Goodwin: We will now continue with experiences of cyproterone acetate and related drugs in the treatment of prostatic disease.

Cyproterone Acetate Treatment of Disseminated Prostatic Cancer and Benign Nodular Hyperplasia

W. W. Scott

Hopkins Hospital, Baltimore, Maryland, USA

My assignment this morning is to present our experience with cyproterone acetate in treating both disseminated prostatic cancer and benign nodular hyperplasia.

Our laboratory experience began in 1963 when we obtained this steroid from Schering through *Karl Kimbal.* We immediately ran this drug through our rat and dog screens, and were impressed.

For many years, longer than I like to think, we have tested many, many steroidal compounds for their ability to:

(1) inhibit what we call endogenous androgenic action,
(2) exogenous androgenic action.

We normally use 10 groups of animals. We check the state of the animal, that is whether the testis are present or removed; the change in prostatic weight under different compounds of drug and, finally, the ratio of prostatic weight to final body weight, upon which we calculate the index. It must be noted here that cyproterone acetate, in the dosage shown (has 4/10 in raising from 0.5–2.0 mg, every other day) was effective, in the intact rat, in inhibiting the endogenous androgenic activity, and was also effective in inhibiting exogenous testosterone.

We then tested using the "prostatic-fistula" dog. It is the Mason modification of the Huggins' fistula. In 2 dogs there was a rather prompt decrease in inhibition of prostatic secretion, in the pilocarpine stimulated preparation.

As you know this compound is a strong progestational agent. In the acetate form it is effective by mouth and it appears to have neither androgenic nor oestrogenic activity in either the rat or the dog.

In 1965 we obtained permission from the Federal Drug Administation in our country to study this compound in 10 patients. I wish to emphasise that all of these 10 patients had widespread dissemination of their prostatic cancer, as was evidenced by markedly elevated serum acid phosphatase and osseous metastases on X-Ray. Interestingly enough, all of them were grade III histologically, or poorly differentiated prostatic cancer. At any rate, we studied these patients. Our results:

In 5 of the 10 patients there was a decrease in serum acid phosphatase. From a high level it fell to less than 1 Bodansky unit. Our range of normal for serum acid phosphatase is 0.1 to 1.0 Bodansky units. An additional 2 patients showed decrease to near normal, and in 3 patients there was no change. Now there has always been some question as to the significance of a decrease in serum acid phosphatase. In a study run by the Cancer Chemotherapy National Service Centre and consisting of 12 groups of urologists from throughout the country (including most of us here from the States), there were 2 important indices of improvement which seemed to be important in this study:

(1)   a decrease in serum acid phosphatase,

and

(2)   a decrease in the size of the primary lesion, as determined by rectal palpation.

Most of these people showed some decrease in size and consistency of the gland. Most of them gained weight, most of them relief from pain. Not all of them responded, nor did they respond to subsequent castration or oestrogen therapy.

We concluded our study by saying that we sincerely felt, from the results which we had observed, that they were as good as they were with any of the oestrogens, perhaps better, because we did not observe any untoward side effects — in the form of breast enlargement, or sodium retention.

At the present time this compound is being studied in prostatic cancer for both the previously treated patient who has relapsed, and for the previously untreated patient in a double-blind study by Drs. *Brendler, Flocks, Grayhack, Hodges, MacDonald* and *Scott.*

We had hoped to have some results to report at this meeting, but we are not quite that far along. Especially, we need more patients in the untreated group. Hopefully this information will be available next year, and you can make the judgements for yourself.

After this study on prostatic cancer, I thought it might be important to dry this in patients with benign hyperplasia. We got permission to do this in 1966—67, and we studied this drug in 13 patients who had significant prostatic enlargement. The compound was given at a slightly lower dosage than in prostatic cancer — 50 mg per day.

As a result we believe that the urinary obstructive symptoms after treatment with cyproterone acetate were improved in 11 of the 13 patients. Obviously this is somewhat subjective.

We measured flow rates and compared them, before and after treatment. This was simply done by measuring flow in time, and we believe that flow rates were increased in 9 out of the 13.

Residual urines were lessened in the majority of patients undergoing treatment with cyproterone acetate. We also felt that prostatic size was smaller after treatment.

Other evidence of the decrease in size of the glands was to be had on doing cystograms before and after treatment. The filling defect in the bladder base became less after treatment. I might say that we're not impressed with the accuracy of the cystourethrogram in estimating prostatic size. What we did was to estimate the size, and subsequently, at open operation, in many patients, enucleate the gland and make the comparison. We are not impressed with this method of determining prostatic size.

All of these people had biopsies before and during treatment. They were needle biopsies. Our pathologist had no knowledge of the clinical condition of the patient. In 2 there was insufficient tissue for him to make any pronouncement. What he did was to simply measure epithelial height, to depict the change in epithelial height upon treatment. Each individual's epithelium was compared with the previous height, the height before treatment being assigned a value of 100. In the majority there was a decrease in the epithelial height with treatment, which is consistent with the thought that this compound will cause some degree of epithelial atrophy.

After treatment we saw a profound atrophy in the acinar epithelium. Studying the levels of serum testosterone before and after cyproterone acetate treatment, we found a significant decrease. I might say, that in another series of patients which I studied in our hospital, not having benign hyperplasia, a decrease in serum testosterone was almost universal, using this compound. We think that the level of the serum testosterone or the change of the serum testosterone is a good index of whether the patient is taking the drug.

I feel rather confident that one patient who did not take the drug, showed no atrophy of his prostate. Interestingly enough patient No. 6 was one of the 4 patients who complained of impotence during this series. There were 4 who complained of some degree of impotence, following or during the administration of this compound. I'm very much excited with this compound, more so than any we've tried here before, and we're looking forward with great anticipation and pleasure to testing this drug in comparative study against a placebo.

Treatment of Benign Prostatic Hypertrophy with Progestogens including Gestonorone Caproate

R. Nagel

Free University of Berlin, Dept. of Urology, Westend Clinic, Berlin, Germany

Summary: Since 1965 a total of 73 patients with a benign prostatic hypertrophy (BPH) have been treated with various gestagens. Our results indicate that treatment is advisable only for inoperable patients with indwelling catheter and for patients in stage I with nycturia and serious dysurial complaints. The most effective of the progestogens tested proved to be the gestonorone-caproate (DEPOSTAT), which should be injected in a dosage of 200 mg/week, at least during the first weeks of treatment. Using this system, the nycturia decreased and the dysurial complaints improved in 2/3 of the patients with an absence of or very small amounts of residual urine. In a few cases it was possible to remove the indwelling catheter after a longer period of treatment with gestagens.

Despite the advances in modern surgical medicine, a specific conservative treatment of benign prostatic hyperplasia (BPH) continues to be desirable, since surgical treatment cannot be applied in a number of patients while others, even though symptoms are present, do not yet require operation.

In 1965 *Geller* et al [2] were the first to report on very promising results which they had obtained with the depotprogestogen *17-hydroxyprogesterone caproate* (Delalutin, Proluton Depot) in the treatment of BPH.

In 1968 *Vahlensieck* and *Gödde* [5] as well as *Burger* [1] were able to achieve encouraging results in treating BPH with *gestonorone caproate* (Depostat), a considerably more active depotprogestogen.

In 1969 *Scott* and *Wade* [4] published surprisingly good results achieved in 13 patients with the daily administration of 50 mg *cyproterone acetate*.

Since 1965 we ourselves have been treating a total of 73 BPH patients with the following steroids (Fig. 1):

Group 1 (Fig. 2)

20 patients aged 61–81 (average age: 74,5 years) were treated with *17-Hydroxyproesterone caproate* at a dosage of 1 g twice per week. The duration of the treatment was 3–10 months (on an average: 7,3 months).

Results

At the start of treatment 8 out of these 20 patients had been carrying an indwelling catheter (IC) for 2–24 months. These patients were not operable for cardiac diseases. Following treatment over a period of 6 and 10 month, respectively, only 2 out of these 8 patients were able to empty their bladder except for a residual urine amount of roughly 20–30 ml. (Fig. 3)

Fig. 1

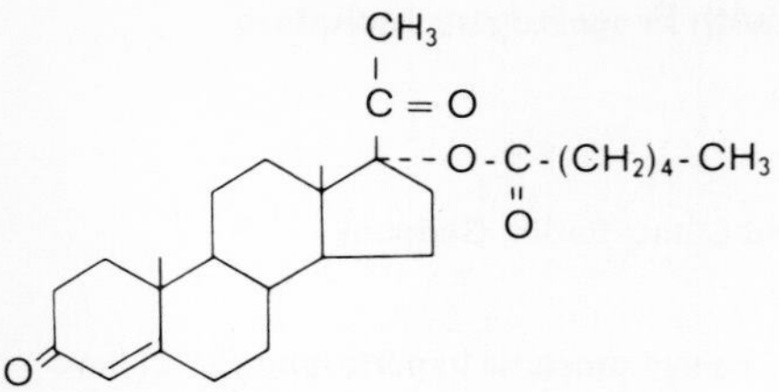

17-alpha-hydroxy-progesterone-
17-caproate (PROLUTON-DEPOT)

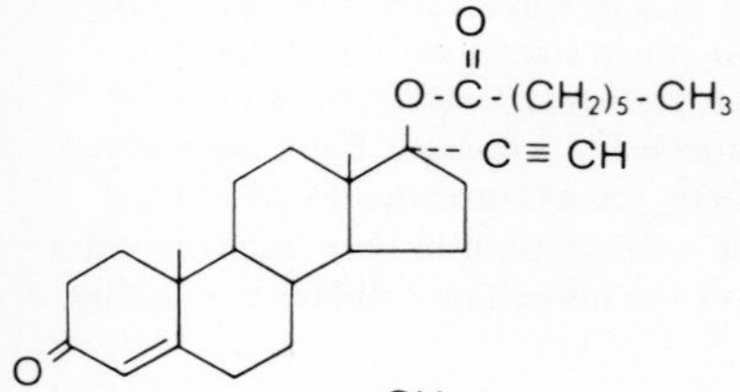

Norethisterone-enanthate

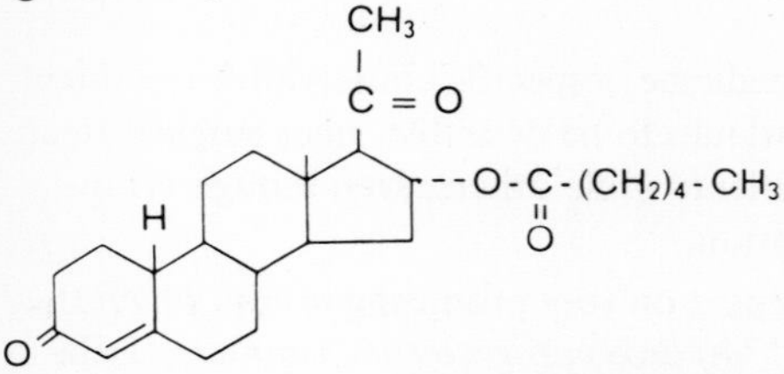

17-alpha-hydroxy-19-norprogesterone-
caproate (DEPOSTAT)

1	No. of patients:	20
2	Age range:	61 − 81 y (mean 74.5)
3	Duration of treatment:	3 − 10 months (7.3)
4	Dosage:	2 x 1.0 g/week

Fig. 2
Group I
17-hydroxyprogesterone-caproate

NO	Age	Duration of treatment (months)	Remarks
1	81	3	No spontaneous mictions. Expired after 3 months
2	73	4	No spontaneous mictions.
3	80	9	No spontaneous mictions. Subjective improvement
4	80	8	No spontaneous mictions. Subjective improvement
5	79	7	No spontaneous mictions. Parkinson's disease
6	80	7	No spontaneous mictions.
7	75	6	RUV 20 ml
8	76	10	RUV 30 ml. Local infiltration

Fig. 3. Group I: 17-hydroxyprogesterone-caproate Patients with indwelling catheters (IC) at start of treatment

The second group involving 12 patients of these 20 did not use an indwelling catheter (IC) at the start of treatment. Only in one out of 4 patients with residual urine volumes between 120 and 220 ml, residual urine decrease to less than 50 ml, while in another patient having 80 ml of residual urine at the beginning of treatment, an indwelling catheter had to be inserted eventually, since residual urine amounts continued to increase. Prostatectomy had to be carried out in another patient because of increasing residual urine. Two patients experienced an acute total retention and could, thereafter, empty their bladder except for slight residual urine amounts. This, however, is well known also to occur without any hormonal treatment. (Fig. 4,5)

From rectal palpation it appeared that the prostate was becoming smaller and firmer in the course of treatment. The distance between internal sphincter and verumontanum which in case of large adenomas was between 5 and 6 cm prior to treatment, as measured by means of the urethroscope, however, did not in any of the cases reveal a significant diminution of the adenoma. Even in larger adenomas this distance was reduced by no more than 0,5—1 cm. Thus all values measured after treatment were within the limit of error and have no significance as to a reduction of BPH.

We can therefore, not confirm the good results obtained by *Geller,* at least as far as this patient group is concerned.

Group 2 (Fig. 6)

Another group of 20 patients aged 62—89 (average age: 70,4 years) was treated with *norethisterone enanthate* over a period of 3—9 months (on an average: 5,5 months). Four patients were injected with 200 mg weekly, whereas 16 patients were given an injection of 200 mg two weeks.

Results·

12 patients were using an IC and only 1 patient was able to empty his bladder except for a residual urine amount of 30 ml after 7 months of treatment.

Another 3 patients were able to empty their bladder in the course of treatment, so that the catheter could be temporarily removed. But TUR or prostatectomy had to be performed on these patients subsequently, owing to renewed increase in residual urine or heavy bleeding.

In those 8 out of the 20 patients without IC at the beginning of treatment whose residual urine was between 30 and 250 ml, no significant reduction in residual urine was observed during 3—9 months of treatment. (Fig. 7).

Thus BPH could not be influenced by this medication.

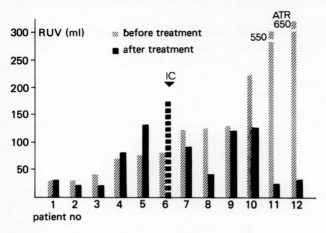

Fig. 4

Group I 17-Hydroxyprogesterone-Caproate 12 pat.

NO	Age	Du — ration of treat — ment (months)	RUV (ml) before treatment	after	Remarks
1	61	4	30	30	Dysuria improved, treatment discontinued
2	73	3	30	20	Dysuria improved, treatment discontinued (heart failure)
3	71	8	40	20	—
4	71	10	70	80	—
5	64	8	75	130	Cardiac insufficiency. Inoperable condition
6	79	7	80	IC	Cardiac insufficiency. Inoperable condition. Subjective improvement
7	87	6	120	90	Local infiltration due to injections
8	75	6	125	40	Diabetes mellitus. Inoperable condition. Dysuria improved
9	61	7	130	120	Prostatectomy
10	74	10	220	120	Cardiac insufficiency. Inoperable condition. Dysuria improved
11	77	7	550(ATR)	20	Local infiltration due to injections
12	81	7	650(ATR)	30	—

Fig. 5. Group I: 17-hydroxyprogesterone-caproate

1	No. of patients:	20
2	Age range:	62 − 89 y (70.4)
3	Duration of treatment:	3 − 9 months (5.5)
4	Dosage:	200 mg/week (4 patients)
		200 mg/every 2 weeks (16 patients)

Fig. 6

Group II
Norethisterone-enanthate

Group 3 (Fig. 8)

This group covered 33 patients aged 56—89 (average age: 72,3 years) with a duration of treatment of 1,5—14 months. (5,0 months on an average).
These patients were given 200 mg *gestonorone-caproate (Depostat)* per week.

Results

10 patients (average age: 79,6 years) were using an indwelling catheter for 2 weeks to 18 months prior to treatment. Spontaneous micturition with residual urine volumes between 20 and 40 ml was brought about in 3 out of these 10 patients. Micturition continued to be satisfactory up to 2 years following treatment.

Another patient was treated with Depostat for 12 months, but micturition resumed only after 6 months' treatment with oestrogens (Progynon-Depot) (Fig. 9).

23 patients aged 56—82 (70 years on an average) without or with only small residual urine volumes up to about 50 ml complained mainly of nycturia and dysuria. Two thirds of these patients, however, experienced substantial improvement of subjective complaints. Dysuria often subsided and nycturia became substantially less pronounced. In 6 patients nycturia had not improved; only regression of dysuria was reported (Fig. 10).

Two thirds of the patients stated that their general well-being had improved substantially and that they felt more energetic. This could, of course, be due to the fact that their sleep was no longer disturbed by nycturia. Other patients, however, without pronounced nycturia also reported that they felt more energetic. A 72-year- old patient complained of a temporary impaired libido.

It is worth mentioning that mainly in the presence of dysuria and nycturia, i.e., in stage I of BPH after roughly 2 months of treatment, one injection of 200 mg Depostat every 2 weeks seems to be sufficient, in order to maintain the therapeutic result achieved at the time. This clinical observation is in accordance with the experimentally determined duration of action of Depostat (3).

Discussion

The *mode of action of* progestogens on the prostate and the adenoma, respectively, is not yet known. In animal experimental studies *Hahn* et al [3] discovered not only an antigonadotropic action of the gestonorone-caproate (Depostat) but also a direct effect on the prostate and seminal vesicles which appears to be independent of the diencephalo-pituitary system. On the basis of our clinical study we ourselves cannot contribute toward answering this question.

As regards the *reduction of adenoma size,* it could be demonstrated through measuring the distance between sphincter internus and verumontanum before and following treatment that there was no significant diminution of this distance in any of the patients, i.e., the diminution of distance was in all cases within the limit of error.

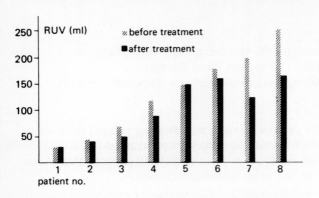

Fig. 7

Group II
Norethisterone-enanthate
8 patients

1	No. of patients:	33
2	Age range:	56 – 89 y (72.3)
3	Duration of treatment:	1.5– 14 months (5.0)
4	Dosage:	200 mg/week

Fig. 8

Group III
SH 582 Gestonorone-
caproate

NO	Age	Du– ration of treat– ment (months)	Remarks
1	82	14	After 16 months RUV 40 ml, later on temporary IC (4 weeks), since 1 year without catheter, RUV 20-40 ml
2	78	12	No spontaneous miction, IC. TUR after 3 months of treatment
3	78	12	No spontaneous miction, IC; however, spontaneous miction after 6 months of treatment with PROGYNON - DEPOT (100 mg/mo). General condition reasonably improved.
4	81	8	No spontaneous miction, IC; expired
5	89	6	No spontaneous miction, still IC after 2 years of treatment
6	76	6	IC removed after 2 months of treatment. Check-up after 2 years: RUV 20 ml. Transient mammary swelling, general condition good. Expired 3 years after treatment
7	85	6	No spontaneous miction, IC; general condition improved
8	67	5	No spontaneous miction, IC; expired 2 months after cessation of treatment
9	79	5	After 6 weeks RUV 20 ml; general condition improved
10	85	3	No spontaneous miction, IC

Fig. 9. Group III: SH 582 Gestonorone-caproate Patients with indwelling catheters (IC) at start of treatment

No.	Age	Duration of treatment (months)	RUV(ml) before treatment	RUV(ml) after treatment	Nycturia before treatment	Nycturia after treatment	Remarks
1	69	6	-	–	2–3	0–1	-
2	65	6	30	10	3–4	1–2	
3	74	8	30	10	5–6	1–2	Subjective improvement
4	68	6	30	10	1	1	Expired
5	80	10	30	30	4–5	1–2	Expired
6	56	7	30 (ATR)	25	3	1	1 x ATR after 10 months, followed again by spontaneous mictions
7	72	4	40	20	1–2	0–1	Severe dysuria. Free of symptoms after treatment. Temporary impaired potency. Testicular biopsy: normal
8	70	5	50 (ATR)	10	2–3	0–1	Medical check-up after 3 years: exellent condition
9	65	6	50	20	1–3	0–1	Medical check-up after 2 years: definite improvement
10	68	6	50	-	1	0–1	Subjective improvement
11	75	6	80	30	3	0–1	Excellent condition
12	85	3,5	20	20	2	0–1	Subjective improvement
13	56	1,5	10	-	2	0	Subjective improvement
14	70	3	20	-	2–3	0–1	Dysuria improved
15	66	4	25	10	1	1	–
16	59	4	20	10	2–3	0	–
17	82	3,5	(ATR)	40	2	1–2	No change
18	58	3	30	-	2	1	Micturition better
19	80	3	60	60	3–4	3–4	Leukemia. No improvement
20	72	1,5	30	10	3–4	2–3	By pass-op. 1968
21	82	3	10	-	6	2–3	Since 1966 Progynon-Depot; Now much better
22	74	3	25	-	4	1–2	–
23	67	3	40	20	2–3	0–1	Excellent condition

Fig. 10. Group III: SH 582 Gestonorone-caproate Patients with predominant dysuric complaints

It is noteworthy, however, that on rectal palpation the prostate was found to have become smaller and firmer in almost all cases. Under the influence of Depostat there is obviously a regression of the accompanying congestion which is present in the majority of cases.

In our view, the fact that individual patients after removal of the IC were able to empty their bladder satisfactorily, in the course of Progestogen treatment, and that in some cases residual urine was reduced to values below 50 ml should not in any case be overestimated.

On the grounds of our hitherto gained clinical experience and as significant side effects have not been observed so far, we think there are only two indications for the treatment of the BPH with Depostat:

1. Inoperable patients with an IC
2. Patients in stage I of BPH, without residual urine, suffering mainly for dysuria and nycturia or patients in the very beginning of stage II with very small, non-infected residual urine volumes and dysuria who either in principle or for the moment refuse the recommended operation.

On the basis of our clinical results we cannot in any case agree with *Burger* in whose opinion " the results obtained with gestonorone caproate (Depostat) were so encouraging that surgery may in the near future be eliminated in a large percentage of cases"; neither we can confirm the favourable results obtained with 17-hydroxy-progesterone caproate (Delatulin) by *Geller* et al. But we think that there is a place for progestogens in the conservative treatment of BPH at least in a certain group of patients as mentioned.

References

[1]   *Burger, A. J. S.:* The management of prostatism. Med. Proc. **14**, 116 (1968).

[2]   *Geller, J., Bora, R., Roberts, Th., Newman, H., Lin, A.* and *Silva, R.:* Treatment of benign prostatic hypertrophy with hydroxyprogesterone caproate.
J. amer. med. Ass. **193**, 121 (1965).

[3]   *Hahn, J. D., Neumann, F.* and *Berswordt-Wallrabe, R. von:* Tierexperimentelle Untersuchungen mit 19-Nor-17-hydroxy-progesteron-capronat (Gestonoroncapronat) im Hinblick auf eine mögliche therapeutische Anwendung beim Prostataadenom, Urologe **7**, 208 (1968).

[4]   *Scott, W. W.* and *Wade, J. C.:* Medical treatment of benign nodular prostatic hyperplasia with cyproterone acetate. J. Urol. (Baltimore) **101**, 81 (1969).

[5]   *Vahlensieck, W.* and *Gödde, St.:* Behandlung der Prostatahyperthrophie mit Gestagen. Münch. med. Wschr. **110**, 1573 (1968).

W. E. Goodwin: Some years ago, Dr. *Kaufman* and I made a somewhat similar study in which, at the suggestion of Dr. *Huggins,* we used a mixture of 20 mg of testosterone and 1 mg of stilboestrol to treat people with benign hypertrophy. We also thought we observed the prostate becoming firmer and the residual urines less, but we weren't sure whether this was a specific effect[3].

[3] *Kaufman, J. J.* and *Goodwin, W. E.:* Hormonal Management of the Benign Obstructing Prostat: Use of Combined Androgen-Estrogen Therapy. The Journal of Urology **81**, 165–171, January 1959.

Use of cyproterone acetate in stages III and IV

G. R. Nagamatsu: This is a report on 22 patients with prostate carcinoma, grades III and IV, which we have studied for 4 years, using cyproterone acetate. 12 of these cases were in the "untreated" category, and 10 were in the "previously-treated" category. 8 cases are stage III and 4 are stage IV in the former group; and 4 and 6 (in stages in III and IV resp.), in the latter group.

All these cases were proven by biopsy. All had endocrine studies, chest x-rays, biopsy of prostate and other data. This was started 4 years ago and the clinical data on actual patients were not clearly elucidated at that time.

The effect of this drug on pituitary-adrenal function was assayed, and our results agree with others, namely that there is no substantial primary effect of this drug in these areas. Control studies under metapyrone stimulation were performed, and no untoward results were recorded.

Testosterone plasma levels were determined using the double isotope method of *Riondel.* Significantly, the reported findings are at castration levels. These studies must be performed under carefully controlled laboratory conditions. Also, the time of collection of the specimen must be the same for all samples because of the wide swing in levels diurnally.

I would like to stress that in not one of these cases, serious side effects were noted. Gastric distress was the most frequent complaint, in the form of heartburn or a little distress after meals. Superficial thrombophlebitis of several days duration was noted in one case, localized to one area. In this susceptible age group, this is a common finding and whether or not this was related to the drug, one cannot say. There was no breast enlargement, no fluid retention, no effect on cardiac function.

In three cases glucose tolerance was definitely decreased. Although the patients are in the category where diabetes of the arteriosclerotic variety can develop, this complication is probably drug related. In some ways the mechanism of action of cyproterone would partially explain this disturbance in glucose tolerance. Daily oral administration of orinase was sufficient for control, and parenteral methods were not required.

The length of administration of cyproterone acetate varied from a maximum of 3 years, 5 months to a minimum of 5 months. Only two patients had the drug for less than one year. The length of temporary improvement varied from as little as three months to as long as over two years. In the previously treated category, ten patients were at the end of stage III or perhaps approaching stage IV. Consequently, this series was a severe test of the drug relative to the stage of the disease. In the stage IV cases, the drug was used as a last effort, and temporary improvement was noted in four of these advanced cases. The length of improvement was mostly subjective. Very few of the objective parameters were altered in this group. The length of subjective improvement and some of the objective parameters varied from as little as three to four months to as long as about one and one half years.

One case is worthy of reporting because of its complete change in the usual clinical behavior: In 1959 an enlarged benign prostate was removed by open surgery. Six years later he appeared with an advanced carcinoma of the prostate, forming a complete fixed rock hard shelf as noted by rectal palpation. Review of the previous slides showed no evidence of neoplastic cells. Castration followed by estrogens was performed according to the standard procedure. However, the prostate did not resolve in size and consistency as is usual with this type of management. Ten months later, the prostate was larger with impending retention, and he was started on cyproterone acetate, 250 mg. a day. Four months later there was a marked decrease in the alkaline phosphate, but the acid phosphatase was up to 5 units. The medication was well tolerated, and by July 1966, ten months after institution of cyproterone therapy, there was a marked reduction in size of the prostate. A recent complete study disclosed a small soft prostate and the acid phosphatase had dropped to 1.5 units. He is one of the patients who developed diabetes. His blood sugar started to rise after two years of treatment and the fasting sugar went up to 160 mg %, and is now up to 200. Clinically he is faring well, requiring only oral medication for control.

In summary, we feel that this drug is worthy of further investigation. Secondly, this does have a real biological effect on the tumor. Thirdly, there is evidence beginning to come forth that it does have a salutory effect in certain cases of grade III, and in some instances, at least subjectively on grade IV tumors.

Cyproterone therapy in stage IV

R. B. Smith: We began studying cyproterone acetate in 1966 and felt that since carcinoma of the prostate is such a difficult disease to really assess in an accurate way, we should pick the most difficult group of patients that is those with stage IV carcinoma of the prostate, who had been on oestrogen therapy, and have either shown no effect or have relapsed during therapy. Since 1966 we have treated 35 patients in this group.

Figure 1. This is the age range of the patients on whom we used the drug along with the racial distribution, which did not seem to have any effect on the progession of their disease.

Figure 2 shows the length of time since the patients were diagnosed as having carcinoma of the prostate, prior to our changing them to cyproterone therapy.

Figure 3. These are the sites of metastatic spread in our 35 patients. The majority of them had bony and soft metastases in the distribution that you see there. Three patients were admitted to the study because they had hydronephrosis, secondly to periureteral spread of their carcinoma.

Figure 4. These were the prior forms of therapy that these patients had been on. You notice that 35 patients were in the study and one patient had *not* been given previous stilboestrol therapy for any length of time. This patient is quite interesting because he could not tolerate stilboestrol owing to congestive heart problems, no matter how energetically he was treated with known modalities of treatment for congestive failure. I might say that he was placed on cyproterone acetate, a dose of 300 mg a day, which was the dosage schedule which we have used. He had no difficulty whatever tolerating this drug.

Fig. 1. Age range and racial distribution

Age

Range	38–82 years
Mean	66.9 year

Race

Caucasian	27
Negro	7
Oriental	1

Fig. 2. Duration of time from initial diagnosis

3–6 months	7
Less than 1 year	8
Less than 2 years	4
Less than 3 years	5
Less than 4 years	3
Less than 5 years	4
Over 5 years	3

Fig. 3. Site of metastatic spread

Bone	31
Soft	
Lung	5
Supraclavicular	3
Liver	3
Penis	1
CNS	1

Periureteral spread with hydronephrosis   3

Fig. 4. Prior forms of therapy

Stilbestrol	34
Orchiectomy	33
Transurethral resection	24
Stilphosterol (I. V.)	6
Radiation Rx	7
Subtotal prostatectomy	2
Radical prostatectomy	2
Cryoprostatectomy	1
^{32}P	1

Fig. 5. Main symptoms

Bone pain		25
Improved	12	
No change	7	
No follow-up	6	

    Duration of improvement: 1, $1\frac{1}{2}$, 3, 4, 6*, 8, 10, 15, 18*, 20, 24*, 24* months

Weakness		15
Improved	5	
No change	8	
No follow-up	2	

    Duration of improvement: 3, 4, 6*, 8, 10 months

Hydronephrosis		3
Improved	2	
No change	1	

    Duration of improvement: 18* and 30* months

Fig. 6. Residual urine

Initial

Less than 20 cc	17
20–40 cc	5
40–70 cc	2
Greater than 70 cc	8
Recent TUR or urethral stricture	3

Effect of SH 714

Improved	6
No effect	7
No follow-up	2

Figure 5. These are the main symptoms with which these patients presented to us. 25 patients had bone pain, and on a dosage schedule of 300 mg a day, we noted an improvement in 12 of these patients. Now underneath you see the duration of improvement. These numbers are in months. Those numbers that have a star next to them are patients still on treatment and still in remission from this particular symptom. This table was made approx. 6 mos. ago. All patients, throughout the whole series of tables, who have a star, are still in remission. So you can add 6 mos. to those values which you see on the tables.

As far as weakness and debilitation from their carcinoma of the prostate is concerned we noted improvement in 5 patients. The duration is noted there. The hydronephrosis was dramatic. In 2 patients there was a complete reversion of their pyelograms to normal. One patient had non-function of one kidney and to this day —35 mos. after the start of treatment — he has a normal pyelogram.

Figure 6. The residual urines were determined and seventeen patients surprisingly had what we considered normal residual urines. Among the patients with residual urines greater than 20 ccs., six patients were noted to have improvement, seven patients had no effect and there wasn't an adequate follow-up in two patients. Three patients who had a recent transurethral resection, or had urethral stricture, were excluded from this determination.

Figure 7. The change in prostatic size, in our experience, was quite dramatic in several patients. We noted a definite decrease in size in twelve of our patients. Sixteen had no change that we could assess. I must say that in the group of 12, there were about 5 patients who had a profound decrease in their prostatic size. One of the patients whose tumour obstructed his ureters had a gland which I would estimate well over 100 mg in size. I can hardly feel his prostate today and this is 23 mos. after starting therapy.

Figure 8. This shows the effect on the alkaline phosphatase. We had only 15 patients, from our severely metastatic group, who had elevated alkaline phosphatases. We saw some change in that group. There was a decrease in 4 of them. You see the values here, measured in King Armstrong units.

Fig. 7. Change in prostatic size and firmness while on therapy

Decrease in size and firmness	12
No change	16
No adequate follow-up	7

Fig. 8. Alkaline phosphatase

Initial

Normal	16
Elevated	15
Study not done initially	4

Effect of SH 714

Decreased	4	(14.0 to 5.0)
		(18.0 to 10.0)
No change	8	(64.0 to 14.0)
		(14.5 to 5.5)
No follow-up	4	

Figure 9. Only eight patients had elevated acid phosphatase determination at the start of treatment. Values ranges from 5.9 to 30 King-Armstrong units. Three patients noticed decrease in acid phosphatase. These three patients also had dramatic reversal in their clinical course. I might also say that we measured all the parameters that Dr. *Nagamatsu* measured, and we did not find any aberrations I might say that 5 patients in our group had decreased platelet counts (below 100,000) at the time they were put on the drug and in 4 of them, there was an increase in the platelet count up to normal levels. We had one patient who had to be taken off the drug because of a very severe allergic dermatitis. He had no previous allergic history, so to be sure we took him off the drug for a month, and then restarted treatment on him. Indeed, he got the dermatitis again. So I think there's little doubt that we have one case to report of dermatitis as a side effect of the drug.

We did not run glucose tolerance tests on all our patients. We had one patient who did develop clinical diabetes while on the medications, however he has a rather strong family history of diabetes, and he's in the age group where you'd expect him to get this, so it's not clear whether you can relate this to cyproterone or not.

Figure 10. We tried this drug on a group of ten patients whom we considered *really* terminal patients. They were in the last stage of their disease, and we only noted a definite improvement in two of these patients. Two of the patients had very transient improvement. The main improvement that occurred, even though their weakness and debility continued to progress, was some relief in the amount of discomfort due to pain, and thus they were able to case up on their pain medication to some extent. We saw no effect from the cyproterone in six out of these ten extremely ill patients.

Figure 11. We tried to compare the initial response of these patients when they were started on stilboestrol therapy to their initial response on cyproterone. In our group we had six patients with no response either to cyproterone or stilboestrol. Thirteen patients had initial response to both drugs. Three patients had response to stilboestrol, but no response to cyproterone acetate, and six patients had a response to cyproterone acetate only, having absolutely no response to stilboestrol when it was started. Seven patients weren't really on the compound long enough to make an evaluation. I'd like to emphasise what Dr. *Nagamatsu* has said, in that we cannot really say whether the survival was prolonged or not, although in some of the patients, it appears it was. The quality of life that these patients had in the remeining few months or years was dramatically improved. I also want to state that we had five patients besides the one patient who couldn't tolerate stilboestrol, who had severe problems with oedema, but were able to be taken off all diuretic agents, when they were taken off stilboestrol and put on cyproterone acetate. So I think this has a distinct advantage over stilboestrol in the treatment of carcinoma even if it were for this one aspect only. All our patients who had been on stilboestrol had gynaecomastia which was, of course, very troublesome for them. All patients responded and got very great relief from their symptoms of gynaecomastia, within one to two months of switching over to cyproterone acetate.

Figure 12. Shows our overall impression of the drug. These figures do include these 10 terminal patients. Again, carcinoma of the prostate is a very difficult disease to assess and this table includes subjective as well as objective improvement. 19 out of the 28 patients on the drug long enough to follow were improved. In 9 patients we saw no improvement. The duration of improvement is tabulated below, in months. Every patient with a star still experiences improvement. You can add 6 months to each of those figures. So, we are very impressed with cyproterone acetate. We have found very good results in this extremely difficult category of patients to treat. I think it has a real place in the treatment of carcinoma of the prostate.

Fig. 9. Acid phosphatase

Initial

Normal	24
Elevated	8
No information	3

Effect of SH 714

Decreased	3	(12.2 to 0.5)
		(23.0 to 0.9)
No change	3	(30.0 to 12.8)
No follow-up	2	

Fig. 10. Effect in 10 terminal patients

Improved (definite)	2
Improvement (transient)	2
No effect	6

Fig. 11. Comparison of response to stilbestrol and SH 714.

Response to neither	6
Response to both	13
Response only to stilboestrol	3
Response only to SH 714	6

(7 patients not on compound long enough to evaluate)

Fig. 12. Overall impression of the effect of SH 714

Improvement seen	19
No improvement seen	9
No follow-up	6
Taken off (allergic)	1

Duration of improvement in months

1, $1\frac{1}{2}$, 3, 4, 6*, 6,6*, 6*, 8, 10, 15, 18*, 18*, 18, 19, 20, 24*, 30*, 32*

R. J. Veemena: I have no formal presentation, but I can briefly give some of our experience with the SH 714. Our initial work was presented at the last conference on this subject in which Dr. *Nehme* reported on patients treated, who had been previously refractory to other forms of hormonal control treatment. Our experience is similar to that which has been presented this morning. At that time we had no significant complications and we have in our 2nd study investigated 39 patients who had no previous treatment for prostatic carcinoma. There were 36 of these who had what we call "short-term" therapy with SH 714 given for 2 months prior to the orchiectomy. Three of the patients refused orchiectomy, so they cannot be classed specifically as "short-term" cases. 27 have now gone on to a position where we can evalute them in what we call "long-term" therapy for 3 to 42 months.

Taken from the notes of Dr. *Markewitz* and Dr. *Gursel* of the department, I find that our experience parallels that reported to you by Dr. *Scott,* Dr. *Nagamatsu* and Dr. *Smith*. We too have seen effects on pain. I have the figures of all of these, but I won't bore you with them at the moment. It's about the same proportion of patients. I think in one of them we have the effects on prostatic size, and consistency. Also the reduction of hydronephrosis has been seen, and the effects on serum acid phosphatase. For example, in that particular parameter in the 'short-term' therapy, there were 16 of the patients of these 36 that had elevated serum acid phosphatase, and in 15 it was reduced to a normal level. In the 'long-term' therapy, with orchiectomy, there were an additional 7 that were subsequently reduced. So this was the orchiectomy, now, added to the SH 7−14. The effect of prolongation of SH 7−14 still of course remains a question.

Now, one thing I think I should mention. This gives some support to our concern about the diabetes. We did see 6 patients with elevated blood sugars and 3 patients are what we would call diabetics and need to be controlled on the usual diabetic regimens. One of these does have a family history of diabetes but the others, I think are *more* than just coincidental. The other 3 with slightly elevated sugars and poor glucose tolerance can be managed by simple dietary measures alone. One patient who was a diabetic, an additional patient, was started on SH 7−14 for prostatic carcinoma. This did indeed complicate, as we might expect, the internist's problems with the management of his diabetes and the treatment was subsequently discontinued.

One of the reasons why we have 2 groups − 'short-term' and 'long-term' − is the desire of Dr. *Markewitz* and all of us concerned with SH 7−14, to see the effects on the human testis. The patients do undergo a dramatic effect both on the germinal epithelium, and on the leydig cells − and this is in print in Investigative Urology. We have also done follow-up biopsies of the prostate in 14 patients and this proves to be rather interesting, with cup biopsy or needle biopsy when no Ca was found, it of course doesn't prove the carcinoma was *not* present in the prostate. It just means that the biopsy was negative. In 6 out of 10 rebiopsied by 'cupbiopsy', we didn't find the Ca at the second biopsy. Four of the patients needed transurethral prostatectomies for obstructive symptoms and 2 of these had no Ca in the specimens. One of them had 60 g of tissue removed, and the other ± 20 g. These are interesting obervations and we all know their limitations, but I thought I'd add them to this conference.

W. Mauermayer: We have treated a group of 66 patients with cyproterone acetate. The dose was 200 mg a day. The study was started 2 years ago. All patients came to us with advanced cancers of the prostate, Grade III and IV. Most of them needed a TUR for relief of obstruction. Eight patients were taken out of the study because they had received oestrogens from their family physicians. Twenty patients died, and it's remarkable that the deaths occurred during 1st treatment. They did not respond to cyproterone acetate, nor did they respond to any other therapy either, which was started when we noticed bone metastases during treatment. They responded to no drug treatment whatsoever.

Now, I'll speak about the group still under observation. The largest group is the group with 2 years treatment, but we have treated 7 patients for 4 years, and one for 5 years. Our general impression is that the compound is affecting the patient in a way that we have not seen before. Impressive, was the gain of weight, the increase of appetite, and an improvement in general feeling of well-being. Veteran patients could be made ambulatory. Some patients remain in this stage despite extensive bone metastases. There were no side effects such as effeminisation, gynaecomastia or oedema. Our experience of 5 years justify a continuation of this study.

P. Mellin: 20 patients with a carcinoma of the prostate group IV (with metastases in lymphonodi and bones) were treated with 300 mg Cyproteroneacetate daily. 13 of them had undergone an estrogen-therapy previously without success, 7 persons were untreated. Only 3 of 20 patients showed objective signs of a temporal limited improvement so as regression of osseous metastases or drop of elevated acid phosphatases. They belonged to the group of cases who did not respond to estrogen-therapy. On the other hand there were 2 previously untreated patients who developed a marked growth of the tumor under cyproteroneacetate therapy, and they did better after administration of estrogens. Surprisingly a high rate of patients, three of twenty, developed paraplegias after spontaneous fractures of vertebrae due to metastases. None of the twenty lived longer than 14 months.

In spite of the poor results almost all patients had the impression of a better general feeling and a relief of pain during the first time of treatment with cyproterone acetate. We feel this compound may be an aid in a limited number of cases when estrogens fail.

High dosages of stilboestrol

W. E. Goodwin: Dr. *Elmer Belt* wishes to tell us his view about large doses of stilboestrol.

E. Belt: This is not so much my view as my experience. Early in our use of stilboestrol we began using high dosages of stilboestrol, largely because of reports of the effectiveness at high level dosages which came out of England. So, we began to use 100 mg 3 times a day — 300 mg a day. This was well-tolerated if taken with food. When we started out using the smaller dosage, at the very first introduction of this drug, we noticed a great deal of peripheral oedema — of the lungs and the legs. There was a large gain in weight which we didn't succeed in reducing with diuretics, but in those same patients when we increased the dosage to 100 mg 3 times a day, a very marked change took place. There was not only the fact that these people did not get oedema. Oedema would disappear rapidly when the dosage was increased, and they went back to their normal weight again, but also concurrently they were able to walk upstairs without breathlessness — the oedema of the lungs having disappeared — and they changed in colour. Now a change in colour also occurred when stilboestrol in smaller dosages was given. These patients turned a sort of a lemon yellow, which all of you have seen. They became apathetic: When the dosage was increased, this lemon yellow disappeared, their apathy disappeared and they could become sunburnt once more. On the low dosage the patients wouldn't sunburn. We have a lot of sunshine out in California, and people like to get sunburnt in the summer. They think they look better. These people could not get sunburnt, but on the high dosage they became sunburnt. Now this was also true of the castrates. If you took the testicles off of a man, he became apathetic, sluggish and didn't sunburn. If you added a low dosage of stilboestrol to this, you had the same effect, but if you give these people a high dosage of stilboestrol (300–500 mg), they pick up in energy and they become sunburnt. These are direct observations – they're not opinions. So, we began to use 100 mg of stilboestrol routinely, unless the patient developed nausea, or other things which the stilboestrol caused – unpleasant symptoms. I wrote to *Charlie Huggins* about this, and I got back one of his laconic answers. He said that he would venture to suggest that you would find the 300 mg of stilboestrol in the urine.

Indicator of oestrogen effect

R. Hohenfellner: The fossa of the urethra has basal and superficial cells. The superficial cells are the big ones and the basal cells are the small ones. Normally the incidence of superficial cells is very low, up to 15 %. The incidence rises after oestrogen medication. The incidence of superficial cells is an indicator of oestrogen saturation. According to our experience there is a direct correlation between clinical course and superficial cell incidence.

Castration results in a significant rise in the superficial cells. The choice of the oestrogen preparation and its dose varies individually regarding superficial cell increases, which has proved to be a decisive indicator. According to our experience, increases of superficial cells of 60 % and more, are satisfactory.

Steroids in urine under gestagen

J. Frick: The idea for this study was to investigate the function of the prostate. We made this study in 1967. We gave a gestagen produced by Merck called Gestafortin (= Chlormadinone acetate). We administered 120 mg a week for 5 weeks, and then we measured the steroids in the urine, before, 5 weeks after, and 8 weeks or longer after the treatment.

We checked 21 patients. There was no change before, after 5 and after 8 weeks of treatment. Also there was no change in the pregnandiol. There was no effect on the gonadotrophins, nor on the 17-keto steroids, nor on the 17-hydroxy ketosteroids.

The oestrogens showed a remarkable increase 8 weeks after treatment. The citric acid in the blood also showed, after 5 weeks, a remarkable increase. About 8 weeks after the treatment, the citric acid in the blood dropped down again, very slowly. With this low dosage which we gave, we saw the same subjective changes which were reported by others, but we didn't see any remarkable changes in the urinary steroids. At that time we didn't have our plasma testosterone method going, but now I think that we can get much more accurate data, if we measure the plasma testosterone level in all these patients.

Hormone dependency of the tumor

M. Kramer: I'm not a clinician and it might be allowed me to make a few comments on the basic principles of the therapy of prostatic cancer. Any therapy of prostatic cancer is based upon the assumption that the tumour is hormone dependent. That means that the tumour is *Androgen* dependent. The goal of the existing therapeutic measures is therefore to eliminate the endogenous testosterone production, or in addition, the inhibition of the testosterone action. The testosterone production can be reduced if the testes are taken out by surgical measures. Endogenous testosterone synthesis is inhibited by substances which block gonadotrophin secretion. This is the primary action, for example, of diethyl stilboestrol. If oestrogen therapy has no effect on tumour growth, the reason for the failure of this therapy has to be studied. This can be done by the determination of the serum testosterone levels. If these levels are still low, one might conclude that the tumour has become testosterone independent. If testosterone levels are high, one should determine the gonadotrophin excretion in the urine. In case of normal gonadotrophin excretion, the hypothalamic receptors might have become insensitive to stilboestrol, or the dosage might be too low. – In this case one could increase the dose, or switch over to another oestrogen – for example ethinyl oestradiol, or a progestational agent, which blocks the gonadotrophin secretion too. If the gonadotrophin secretion is low, but the testosterone level is high, which might be the case under long lasting oestrogen therapy, testosterone is derived from other sources – for example, from the adrenals. In this case it might be useful to try an anti-androgen, like SH 714, in order to inhibit the testosterone activity.

Panel Discussion

Participants:

H. Brendler — W. Brosig — R. H. Flocks — C. V. Hodges — J. J. Kaufman —
G. T. Mellinger — W. W. Scott

Moderator:

W. E. Goodwin

W. E. Goodwin: We have a list of questions which we have studied, and I will pose the questions to the panel.

Hormone dosage

The first question we are going to ask Dr. *Scott,* Dr. *Mellinger* and Dr. *Brendler.* It has to do with hormone dosage.

Do different types of drugs make any difference? That is, do different types of oestrogens have different effects?

W. W. Scott: Well, I think that the vast majority of people in the United States would use diethylstilboestrol, in a dosage of 5 mg per day, or less. I think that a dosage of 1–3 mg of diethylstilboestrol is adequate. There are other oestrogens used. We have used Honvan. We have used Tace. The dosage for Tace is two 12 mg capsules daily. The naturally occurring oestrogen Premarin®, which is sodium oestrone sulphate, comes in dosages of 0.6, 1,2 and 2.5 mg. I would say that we would use a total dosage of about 2.5 mg per day. We would either give it in one tablet or three. The long acting oestrogens have not enjoyed too much usage, at least in Baltimore

W. E. Goodwin: We would like to ask if Dr. *Mellinger* has anything to add on this matter of dosage.

G. T. Mellinger: Most of the cardio-vascular problems which we have had in using oestrogens have been at the dose of 5 mg. In the study where we compared 5 mg with 1 mg, and placebo, you will notice that we did not have any trouble to speak of using the 1 mg per day.

W. W. Scott: I have a question for Dr. *Brendler,* as he was the one to analyse the data. Are there any data at all from a double blind study done 10 years ago, where 5 mg of diethyl stilboestrol per day was compared with 500 mg per day, in terms of cardiovascular disease?

H. Brendler: No. We were not aware at that time of the possible hazards in the use of stilboestrol. The study, you will recall, was confined to patients who either had a relapse following castration, or prior oestrogen therapy, and to those who had proven refractory to these measures from the outset. So I have no information for you on that specific point. As for my own opinion concerning the proper dosage of oestrogen, which oestrogen to use and what the treatment regime should be – I can only agree with Dr. *Scott's* feeling on this. We use 5 mg a day, and we have not been aware of any side effects of a vascular nature. I'd be inclined to agree that smaller dosage would suffice, but I must say we've been using 5 mg a day.

W. E. Goodwin: Dr. *Flocks,* do you have anything to add about the type of drug? I know that in the past you were interested in the diphosphate.

R. H. Flocks: One of the interesting things about these drugs, in my experience, has been that a patient who has had an orchiectomy and who becomes refractory to one type of oestrogen (let's say the synthetic diethyl stilboestrol) will frequently get another remission on using a natural oestrogen. We also found in approximately one-third of the patients who have become refractory after orchiectomy and oestrogen (both natural and synthetic) that large doses of Honvan over a period from 10-20 days produce a remission of varying length, sometimes several months, sometimes even as long as 6 months. This is given in intermittent doses of 1 mg daily for 5 days in every month. They continue to do well for several months and then become refractory again.

W. Staehler: As to the results of Dr. *Mellinger,* I believe this is a question of the dosage; in Europe we have a preliminary treatment during the first weeks of much higher doses than I have seen here. The dose is 500 mg. of oestrogens dayly. I think that Dr. *Mellinger's* results including placebo series are explained by this. If you give a small dose in the beginning, resistance develops quickly. If you use a large dose in the beginning, the acid phosphatase falls to zero, whereas if you give small doses, the acid phosphatase does not fall at all or only slightly. It must fall, though, to zero. Thus in the early stages in which oestrogens are used this is of importance. The results are as shown. We think it necessary to begin with a high dose.

As to cardiovascular diseases, we know from the investigations of *W. D. Germer* (Dtsch. med. Wschr. **73**, 280, 1948) that if you give barbiturates during therapy with oestrogens, considerable oedema results. We know this and therefore we don't give barbiturates.

I still continue using oestrogens, and we only see in 2 % of the cases resistance developing early.

Sexual potency after total prostatectomy

W. E. Goodwin: The question of sexual potency after total prostatectomy has been raised. We heard this morning from Dr. *Belt* that 10 % of his patients were able to have an erection. I would like to ask Dr. *Flocks* about those undergoing radical retropubic prostatectomy. How many patients are able to have an erection?

R. H. Flocks: All my patients after radical prostatectomy, both retropubic and perineal, have been impotent.

W. E. Goodwin: Has anyone on the panel had patients who have had normal sexual activity or normal intercourse after total prostatectomy?

H. Brendler: Not normal sexual activity, but some have had erections. I have, from time to time, seen patients who said they've had erections.

W. E. Goodwin: I have seen one of mine who has had erections. We've heard from Dr. *Bagshaw* that 1 in 4 who are treated by irradiation become impotent. I wonder if anyone could explain that.

W. W. Scott: I am not at all certain as to the cause of impotence. From experience, it seems that in transverse, complete ruptures of the urethra, the patient is almost always impotent. *Frank Phifer* who used to do a great many perineceal prostatectomies in Chicago, always used to say that the more he enlarged the perineum dissection to expose the prostate to the gallery, the greater the chance of the patient being impotent. I presume this would disturb the perineal nerves. Of course, some of this is above the collar, because I have been told by two patients, post-castration and on oestrogen, that they were not impotent. Well, this is pretty good, if it is true. So I don't know what irradiation would do, unless it caused damage to the nerves. I would not know any other mechanism.

W. E. Goodwin: Dr. *Hodges,* do you have anything to add to that?

C. V. Hodges: Well, I would think, also, it must be caused by injury to the nerve supply. I can not think that the arterial supply would be stenosed by irradiation. That would be the other possibility.

J. J. Kaufman: I wanted to say something about potency. We have seen sporadic potency, particularly in individuals who are in the 40–50 age group. Of course, we don't have many individuals in that age group, but those that we do have seem to hold on to some measure of potency. What I wanted to stress was that Dr. *Pearman* in our Clinical Faculty at UCLA has had a wide experience (some 80 cases) of placing silastic implants in the penis for organic impotence, and the patients have been very satisfied with this baculum or rib-like prosthesis, which is placed under the tunica albuginea of the corpus and acts as a rod in the penis. As I say, over 80 patients, and from what I can gather, the vast majority are very happy with this. Some of the wives are extremely happy with it. That is just something for the patients who are impotent and want to continue their sexual life.

Incontinence following radical prostatectomy

W. E. Goodwin: We come back to the question of incontinence. We heard this morning that we can expect a 10 % incontinence incidence but there are also some things which have been devised to try to lower this figure. I wonder if Dr. *Flocks* would like to speak on this? What experience have you had with incontinence and what can you say about ways of preventing it?

R. W. Flocks: Incontinence following radical prostatectomy depends a great deal, in my experience at least, on the size of the lesion, and the extent to which the bladder neck and the urethra need to be dissected to get at the carcinoma. If there is a very small lesion, where the entire membranous urethra and possibly the urethra as it enters the apex of the prostate is undisturbed, and if at the same time the bladder neck can be as beautifully dissected as Dr. *Belt* showed us a few minutes ago, and an accurate apposition of the bladder neck to the urethra achieved, incontinence is very infrequent. On the other hand, if the lesions are large, and a good deal of dissection of the trigone is necessary, and if apposition is not adequately secured, either by the retropubic or the perineal route, incontinence is more frequent.

W. W. Scott: In Brady, between 1904–1966 I think, the incontinence rate was 11.8%, but this included all patients operated upon by resident staff and so forth. Dr. *Jewett* who is responsible for the most recent manuscript from Brady on the 15-year survivorship following total perineal prostatectomy, published in one of the January issues of the JAMA for 1969, states that in his last 78 personal cases he has caused no incontinence.

W. E. Goodwin: If the patient is incontinent there are some curative operations that have been devised. We won't spend a great deal of time on this, but it is true that Dr. *Kaufman* has devised the most recent one, and has some most interesting experiences. I wonder, Dr. *Kaufman,* would you take a moment to explain this to us?

Surgical treatment of incontinence

J. J. Kaufman: I'll try to do that very briefly. This is certainly a very preliminary report of an operation which is based on the same premise as the Berry procedure, and more recently the Hinman procedure. Namely, that of upward compression of the bulbous urethra, or the urethra just distal to the bulb, with elevation of the uro-genital diaphragm by some type of implement, will result in the restoration of continence, which is lost following prostatectomy whether transurethral, perineal, suprapubic, or retropubic. As a result of our disenchantment with the Berry operation the patients relosing their continence after a while, loosening of the prosthesis in many of them, draining sinuses, painful perineum, difficulty in sitting down, etc., and because the Hinman operation has not worked out particularly well in our hands (that being, namely, the implantation of a piece of autologous rib across the pelvis, anchoring it to the ischial tuberosity with screws) — we decided to employ another means, which I will now demonstrate with the next few slides. There have been a number of operations employing the use of the ischial cavernosus muscles, which have either been crossed or imbricated. A number of operations have used the bulbo-cavernosus muscles, which lie over the bulb of the penis, but we think that the use of the crus as a compressing device is new. This is a drawing to show the attachments of the crura to the inferior pubic arch, down to this point. Now the ischio cavernosus muscle comes down on the inside of the crus and attaches down here somewhere.

First the crus of the penis is freed. The attachment of the ischial cavernosus to the ischium is ligated. After freeing these crura, they are crossed and attached to the periosteum of the opposite pubic ramus. These crura can be attached at any level to the inferior pubic arch where they make a comfortable apposition.

The incision we use has been called the Mercedes Benz incision, but a perineal incision can be used and it is simply higher. It comes to the base of the scrotum. Actually, it should be a little bit higher than this. It starts over the ischial tuberosities.

The bulb is not molested in any way. By simply retracting laterally on the perineum, the white aponeurotic appearance on the ischial cavernosus muscle can be seen. The crus which is very firmly adherent to the bone, is removed now. If the bone is "hugged" by the scissors, it will save cutting into the tunica albuginea of the crus.

The opposite ischial cavernosus muscle is exposed. When the two ischial cavernosus muscles and crura have been freed on both sides, we appose this crus to the opposite side, where it is attached with heavy silk to the inferior pubic arch.

One crus is crossed over here, the other is crossed under, and one suture is taken in the middle.

W. E. Goodwin: What is the suture material?

J. J. Kaufman: 00 or 0 silk. The operation is extremely simple. We have done a total of 12 of these operations. The shortest follow-up is approximately 6 hours, and as far as I know he is still continent. The longest follow-up is roughly 5 months. It remains to be seen whether these patients will maintain their continence, which is present to a 100 % degree. Rather I would say to something slightly less than 100 % degree, as the I'st two patients have stress incontinence, which is probably due to the fact that I did not tighten them enough. Whether the corpora will become fibrotic or not, we don't know. This might cause some late failure after an early success. The patients complain of some numbness of the scrotal skin and penis, which is attributable to cutting a few branches of the pudendal nerve. The sensation is regained after a month. Sexual function is difficult to assess in these patients, because our average age is 70. But one man told me that it was not quite as good, for instead of having a semi-annual erection, he now is having an annual semi-erection. We don't know about potency.

Prevention of incontinence

W. E. Goodwin: I'll ask Dr. *Brendler* a question on technique: It has been said that there was less chance of continence if you left a little bit of apical tissue when you cut across the urethra. I wonder if you have any experience with this, or any opinion about it?

H. Brendler: I have not had any experience with this. I can simply report to the audience that this has come to my attention. I have met a number of urologists who utilise the perineal approach for total prostatectomy and who have expressed the opinion, that when the carcinoma is situated in the upper portion or base of the prostate, and where they felt reasonably certain that the apical portion of the prostate was free of carcinoma, that it is feasible to leave the apex of the prostate behind with the idea that the patient can be more assured of total urinary continence. I don't do this, so I don't advocate it, I simply report this to the audience, and I would personally appreciate the opinions of other members on the panel.

J. J. Kaufman: Well, I don't think it is necessary to preserve a piece of the prostate. I'd do it in total prostatectomies for non-carcinomatous conditions, such as calculous disease. An important point in either the retropubic or the perineal operation is to incise just at the apex of the prostate to get a few of the fascial fibres which will allow you to lengthen the urethra. Just above the membranous urethra there is a portion of the urethra, which is almost intussuscepted, as it were, into the apex of the prostate.

You get more length, and then you have a good 1 1/2 to 2 cm of urethra to use. I doubt very much whether continence is related directly to leaving the apex of the prostate behind or not, provided you have not traumatised the urogenital diaphragm.

Radical prostatectomy and orchiectomy

W. E. Goodwin: I am going to ask Dr. *Hodges* a question. If you do a radical prostatectomy for cancer, do you also do an orchiectomy? If so, when? Under which circumstances?

C. V. Hodges: I can not recall doing any orchiectomy at the same time as a radical prostatectomy. I believe that if one wants to find out whether a radical prostatectomy is going to be effective in controlling cancer, one can not, at the same time, employ other measures—either orchiectomy or oestrogens. So I would only do the radical procedure.

Therapeutic principles in the different stages of prostatic cancer

W. E. Goodwin: Now we'll come back to the question of indications, and I want the panel to look at Dr. *Flocks'* slide. At the top he's got A, B, C, and down below D and E. We use more or less this same schema at UCLA. We consider that A and B are curable by radical prostatectomy and that the others are not, but I'd like to ask the panel. I think we'll just do it at random. We'll start with group A. How do you handle that kind of case, Dr. *Brendler?*

H. Brendler: I have no quarrel with what you've outlined. I think that group A is potentially curable, and should be handled by radical prostatectomy, my own preference being the perineal route.

W. E. Goodwin: Dr. *Scott,* if you have a case like the C, up there, do you think there is a place for giving pre-operative oestrogens to make it shrink and then to try and do a radical prostatectomy?

W. W. Scott: I don't think you can make an inoperable prostatic cancer operable, whether with oestrogen or castration. Dr. *Winfield Wentworth Scott,* formerly Professor at the University of Rochester, New York, is a great advocate of this, and his figures actually look better than the figures for a radical on early lesions. On the other hand they are not graded. In our institution we would handle A by total perineal prostatectomy. I think we would take more of the perivesicular fascia, and more of the bladder neck. I don't know whether this makes any difference, because in our series of nodules, reported in the JAMA, there was no 15 year survival in the presence of cancer that had spread to the perivesicular fascia. There were also no poorly differentiated cancers that survived 15 years.

W. E. Goodwin: Dr. *Hodges,* how would you handle A and C, and by which route, perineal or retropubic?

C. V. Hodges: I would do a perineal on A, because I would like to do an open biopsy of this nodule. Now it is possible that this man has already had a needle biopsy done by someone else, whereupon he arrives for therapy. I would evaluate my indications on his general build and upon his perineum. If he is not too fat, and if his perineum seems wide enough, I would, preferably, do a perineal prostatectomy. Otherwise I would do a radical retropubic, and I think the results would be about the same.

W. E. Goodwin: Is there anyone on the panel who would do a radical prostatectomy on B up there? The little one at the top with positive nodes.

R. H. Flocks: With regard to A, I would do essentially as has been outlined. I'd do a perineal exposure, biopsy, and a radical. Now if this patient was relatively young (let's say under 70 and in good shape — no cardiovascular problems and so forth) I would assume that he could possibly be in group B. About 10 % fall into this group in my experience. I would do a pelvic lymphadenectomy as a second stage operation. I expect in one out of 10 cases to find some positive nodes and expect that this pelvic lymphadenectomy would make some difference to the ultimate prognosis or history of this patient.

With regard to C, if he was under 70, I would plan to go in there and do a total prostatectomy followed by interstitial radiation.

W. E. Goodwin: You said something about age, and that is one of the questions that has been posed. Dr. *Hodges,* do you have any age limit at which you would not do a radical prostatectomy?

C. V. Hodges: In general we don't do them in patients over 70 years of age. Occasionally we see one who is somewhat older, 71 or 72, but who appears younger physically, and we will include him. Generally, though, we set our cut-off date at 70.

W. E. Goodwin: Dr. *Scott,* do you have a feeling about age in relation to radical prestatectomy?

W. W. Scott: I think that I would express it just as Dr. *Hodges* has.

W. E. Goodwin: Now let's come down to groups D and E. Dr. *Mellinger,* how do you handle group D?

G. T. Mellinger: Group D is that which has local spread, that is, spread outside the prostatic capsule, but without distal metastases.

W. E. Goodwin: Well, it has nodes in this case.

G. T. Mellinger: Do you mean pelvic nodes, or distal nodes? If you mean pelvic nodes, I do not consider these as distal metastases. You mean nodes confined to the pelvis?

W. E. Goodwin: Regional metastases.

G. T. Mellinger: I think that these patients would do just as well without treatment, at that time. Later, if and when (and I emphasize *If*) metastases developed, then it would be time to treat. Metastases do not always develop, at least not in 10 years. At least 35–40 % of stage III patients or in this case D patients, do not develop metastates within 10 years.

W. E. Goodwin: Now what about E, where we have evidence of bony involvement as well as local spread?

G. T. Mellinger: If the patient was in pain, and he probably is, I would definitely treat him, and I would give 1 mg stilboestrol.

W. E. Goodwin: Dr. *Hodges,* what would you do for a patient in group E?

C. V. Hodges: Well, like Dr. *Mellinger,* I believe I would not treat him, if he is asymptomatic. If he does have pain, I would also start him on oestrogens, and I prefer 1 mg daily.

W. E. Goodwin: Dr. *Scott,* one of the questions that has been asked is: When do you start hormone treatment? In other words, what are the indications for starting hormone treatment?

W. W. Scott: Although my old professor, Dr. *Huggins,* was a great advocate of early treatment of prostatic cancer with hormones, I would say that at least since 1946 or thereabouts I have advocated delayed treatment, and relied on the appearance of osseous metastases, causing pain and debility.

W. E. Goodwin: But if you saw metastases without pain, would you treat them?

W. W. Scott: I would not treat osseous metastases, if they were not causing any pain – no.

W. E. Goodwin: How about anaemia, with osseous metastases but without pain?

W. W. Scott: This would suggest widerspread replacement of bone marrow with tumour. I probably would do hormone treatment.

W. E. Goodwin: Does anyone else have anything to say?

H. Brendler: I guess I am the only one on the panel who feels this way, from what I gather, but as soon as I find a patient in stage E prostatic carcinoma, I immediately start endocrine therapy. My feeling about this is based on my belief that the withdrawal of the androgenic stimulus, however accomplished, results in cell death, and a slowing down of whatever growth processes (biological processes) are going on in these cells. Even though we are not yet equipped to evaluate the level of activity of these metabolic processes, because of our inadequate knowledge today, nevertheless I believe these cells can escape at any time, even between frequent periodic examinations. I think we owe it to the patient. I have never seen anyone hurt by endocrine therapy. So it is my belief, it ought to be started immediately. My preference is for castration; however, there are those individuals who for one reason or another would prefer to start on oestrogen therapy and so I start it.

W. E. Goodwin: So you would give maximum treatment from the start.

H. Brendler: Right. There are those who prefer to go on oestrogen therapy, in preference to castration. I would agree, if I think that they are reliable patients, who can be trusted to take their medication, and I won't press too hard for castration. A lot of patients lose confidence, or become fearful, and will drift away or neglect their treatment completely. So I won't press the point because I am not completely convinced in my own mind that the combination of castration and oestrogen really does that much better than oestrogen therapy alone, or castration alone.

W. E. Goodwin: I happen to agree with you. I prefer to do castration when the diagnosis is first made, providing it is not a curable case, and then give oestrogens at the same time.

Subcapsular versus total orchiectomy

One of the questions that has been asked is about orchiectomy, as to when it is done. At the same time we can raise the question about subcapsular orchiectomy versus total orchiectomy. Is there any difference? We happen to have an expert on that in the audience. I am going to ask Dr. *Grayhack* to tell us about his experience in this matter.

J. T. Grayhack: Dr. *MacDonald* at the University of Illinois demonstrated that the remaining tunica albuginea had lydic cells present when a sub-capsular orchiectomy was done. We then tested the function of these patients following subcapsular orchiectomy, by giving them 1000 units of chorionic gonadotrophin three times weekly. We demonstrated an increased excretion of androsterone as well as etiocholanolone, which indicated to us that this testicular remnant after intercapsular orchiectomy continued to function. When the remnant was removed there was no response to chorionic gonadotrophin. If you wish to remove all the tissue that can be stimulated by chorionic gonadotrophin, you should do total orchiectomy, as was initially recommended.

Surgical mortality

W. E. Goodwin: Is there anyone on the panel who does subtotal or sub-capsular orchiectomy? No. So it is a consensus that total orchiectomy should be done, when it is done. A question about surgical mortality. I wonder if anyone on the panel, and we'll start with Dr. *Scott,* can tell us about surgical mortality in the Brady series?

W. W. Scott: I truly can't remember.

W. E. Goodwin: I can't either, but my recollection is that it is less than 1 %.

W. W. Scott: I would say that that figure is reasonable. I mean it is no different than a perineal prostatectomy, in our hospital for benign hyperplasia.

W. E. Goodwin: I think it is safer than a simple perineal.

C. V. Hodges: I can not give you any exact figures, but I would agree that the mortality is very low.

W. E. Goodwin: Dr. *Veenema,* can you tell us, from the audience, about the mortality in your retropubic series?

R. J. Veenema: We had no surgical mortality either in the operating room or immediately post-operatively. There was one patient who died, who had an embolus, followed by jaundice, at a time when the halothane problem was before us. That is the only one we had.

W. E. Goodwin: One died, in the hospital, after operation.

R. J. Veenema: Less than 1 % actually.

Cryo-therapy

W. E. Goodwin: A question came up about experience with cryo-therapy. Dr. *Flocks,* I wonder if you can speak on that.

R. H. Flocks: As many of you know, cryo-therapy has been utilised by the group in Buffalo for the treatment of stage E prostatic carcinoma. For relief of obstruction, and with the possibility that some type of antibodies were created in response to the sloughed tissue. These antibodies then might bring about disappearance or resorption of some metastatic deposits. I have not utilised this therapy in the way that it was utilised at Buffalo, but I have exposed the prostate perineally in patients of stage III, and frozen a large portion of it, in order to do studies which might indicate the possibility of some kind of antibody reaction, or immune reaction. In most cases there was a large amount of slough destruction of the local tissue. A good deal of pain occurred in the initial few weeks following the procedure. This, though, was followed by good healing and good repair locally. So, as far as the local destruction of the tissue is concerned, after sloughing through the perineal wound nothing untoward happened. We could not demonstrate any evidence of antibody formation, or any disappearance or change in the metastatic deposits.

Pathological grading of prostatic cancers

W. E. Goodwin: Now. Dr. *Scott,* what about the pathologists grading by cell type?

W. W. Scott: Well, we graded all our prostatic cancers, and when I say *we,* I mean Dr. *William Shelley,* who is our surgical pathologist. He grades them into four grades (roman numerals I to IV) — I think, by and large, two would be enough — one large group of I and II, and one large group of III and IV. In other words, well differentiated adenocarcinoma and poorly differentiated. The criteria used for grading are essentially the same as were presented by Dr. *Mostofi* in his superb lecture. We sincerely believe that grading influences prognosis. There is a great influence on prognosis, no matter what the treatment is, whether it is hormonal or surgical treatment. As to the accuracy of the grading, we published this in Dr. *Stamey's* Journal as an editorial, a few years ago. There were several hundred cases. Dr. *Gerald Murphy* and I went through the slides and graded them, according to the degree of differentiation of the cells, and in 87 % of the cases we agreed as to the grade. There was no overlap of more than 1 grade in the 13 in which we did not agree.

H. Brendler: How does this square with what Dr. *Belt* told us this morning, in his series of cases, where he expressed the opinion that survival was not correlated with histological grade?

W. W. Scott: I am sorry that I was not here this morning. I did not hear the paper, but perhaps you can tell me what was said.

H. Brendler: I don't remember the total number Dr. *Belt* stated, but if I have noted this correctly, in his series of 398 total perineal prostatectomies for prostatic cancer, the histological grade was not correlated with the survival time. Am I right, Dr. *Belt?*

E. Belt: 90 of our patients were not graded. All the rest were. Grading is in progress now and its influence on survival will be reported.

W. E. Goodwin: There is another series from Boston, reported by *Parkhurst, Kerr* and *Leadbetter,* where they showed there was quite a good correlation between grade and survival.

R. H. Flocks: We had approximately 1200 cases in stages C and D as classified in the above figure. In this group of 1200 cases there were approximately 100 odd cases that were alive 15 years after the initial diagnosis, having received varying treatments. We sent 30 slides at random from this group to Dr. *Shelley* in Baltimore to test him. At the same time we sent 20 slides from patients of the same group, but who had died during the first 5 years after their diagnosis had been made. He graded them for us I, II and III. Grade III was highly undifferentiated; II was the average (areas of moderate differentiation, some areas of poor differentiation); and grade I was highly differentiated. About 90 % of those who died within 5 years fell into grade III. On the other hand — in those who lived — only 3 were grade III, the rest of them were all grade II, so that there was a relationship.

W. W. Scott: Dr. *Flocks,* when did you write that you thought prostatic cancers were not gradable?

R. H. Flocks: Before I sent the slides to *Shelley.*

W. W. Scott: O. K., I was not certain. Do you think they are not gradable now?

W. E. Goodwin: He *does* think they are gradable now.

W. W. Scott: O. K. That is what I thought you said.

H. Brendler: The answer to this may lie in the fact that Dr. *Scott's* study was based on careful serial sectioning of entire prostates, whereas it may well be that routine handling of a surgical specimen does not yield the most malignant area. Dr. *Scott* and Dr. *Schirmer* showed very clearly in the chapter that they wrote for Campbell's Urology that the same specimen could contain several areas of varying morphology and degree of anaplasis. This may be the explanation.

W. W. Scott: I think this may very well be true. What we'd attempted to do was to assign the highest grade to what we saw. In other words, one might see well-differentiated inter-acinar cancer, and one might see a poorly differentiated scirrhous cancer. We would assign the scirrhous cancer to grade III, not to I or II. We have already asked Dr. *Flocks,* or someone did, what he would do if he developed a small nodule, which I hope he never does. I heard that he said he would use gold. Now I would like to ask him, if he was so unfortunate as to have a prostatic cancer – would he rather have a well-differentiated adeno-carcinoma, or a poorly differentiated scirrhous one?

H. Brendler: This figure, which I have taken the liberty of showing, is from Dr. *Scott's* article. These four sections were cut from the same prostate and show, clearly, different histological patterns and degrees of anaplasia.

R. H. Flocks: Well, as I indicated, after testing Dr. *Shelley,* which showed conclusively that those who died within 5 years had a very high incidence of grade III lesions, and those who lived 15 years had a very low incidence of grade III lesions – it is quite obvious that I would not want the grade III lesion. I agree whole heartedly with what Dr. *Scott* said.

W. E. Goodwin: I think we've beaten that dog to death.

Radical retropubic prostatectomy following open perineal biopsy

It has been asked whether anyone on the panel who has had experience doing open perineal biopsies, then does radical retropubic afterwards? Does any one wish to speak on that?

C. V. Hodges: I have done this a number of times, as I indicated earlier. One can get a biopsy and realise at that point that because of a narrow perineum, it is going to be very difficult to do a perineal prostatectomy. Much time will be saved if one simply closes, puts the legs down, with the patient in the supine position, and does a retropubic.

J. J. Kaufman: As I indicated earlier today, I still feel that the needle biopsy, with experience can be extremely accurate. I would like to say one word about Mr. *Turner-Warwick's* remark on the hazard of needle biopsy in implanting cancer in the tract. To the best of my knowledge, Dr. *Burkholder* and I reported the second or third such case, and ours was out of an experience of over 1000 cases of needle biopsy of the prostate. I think this is an extremely rare situation. I don't think we really have to consider this a serious liability.

W. E. Goodwin: I'd just like to say one thing about needle biopsy myself. I think it should be reserved for cases who are not going to have a radical prostatectomy. If you have a patient who is a candidate for radical prostatectomy, you'd better get the biopsy by an open method and get a frozen section. That is my personal feeling, which I feel rather strongly about.

R. H. Flocks: There is a problem with the frozen section. Sometimes it is called 'negative' and then it turns out 'positive' later.

W. E. Goodwin: All right. You just go back another day.

At one time you wrote about how easy it was, retropubically, to turn the prostate around and get to the back side of it. Would you enlarge upon that a little bit, Dr. *Flocks?*

R. H. Flocks: If you are planning a retropubic prostatectomy and want a preliminary perineal needle biopsy, it is relatively simple, once you have the retropubic exposure, to divide the pelvic fascia, insinuate your finger between the posterior surface of the prostate and the rectum, and turn the prostate around. You can thus obtain an adequate biopsy. We have done this many times.

Oestrogen, orchiectomy and combined therapy

W. E. Goodwin: The question on oestrogen and orchiectomy has come up already. I just want to hear from Dr. *Scott.* We have already heard that he does not start treatment upon making the diagnosis, unless there are symptoms, but when you have a patient with symptoms, do you prefer to use oestrogens or orchiectomy, and if so, in which sequence and when?

W. W. Scott: Well, statistics to the contrary, I still feel that bilateral orchiectomy does something that oestrogen administration does not do. I would treat the patient with metastases, causing pain and disability, by castration and oestrogen administration, immediate and continuous.

W. E. Goodwin: Does anyone on the panel differ in that opinion?

C. V. Hodges: I would prefer to start with oestrogens. There is an occasional patient, it seems to me, who after a relapse and escape from control by oestrogens, will still show a favourable response to orchiectomy. I think, perhaps, one can thus lengthen the time that control may be achieved by staging these treatments rather than giving them simultaneously.

W. E. Goodwin: I recently saw a man who was 49 years old who had a metastasis in his 10th dorsal spine. It was not very painful, but he had it. I did orchiectomy as primary treatment in that case. One of the questions which ought to be answered (I am not sure that it can be) is:

"What is your opinion – and also what do you think the general opinion in the United States is, as regards the V. A. study, which we heard reported by Dr. *Mellinger?* " I guess we will start with Dr. *Brendler* on that.

H. Brendler: Well, I can't answer that question. I wish I could. It is so easy for a person to be biased, to listen to those opinions which happen to agree with his own personal prejudices. I have the greatest respect for the group which conducted this study. I am not in a position, nor do I ever expect to be, to be able to sit down and evaluate their statistics critically, or as carefully as I would like to, there just is not enough time. One hears many demeaning opinions about it. I think Dr. *Scott* yesterday levelled two criticisms at this study which I think are valid. Apart from that I have nothing further to say.

J. J. Kaufman: I think it is important for the audience to know that the American urologists find themselves in a very uncomfortable dilemma over this question of hormonal therapy. At the present time, it only permits a very arbitrary decision on the part of the urologist, in regard to the treatment of his individual patient. Everything was nice and clear some 25 years ago when *Nesbitt* and *Baum* came out with what was purported to be a statistically significant study, showing that people lived longer with orchiectomy and oestrogen, than either of these modalities alone, or with nothing. Then there were a number of subsequent papers (a number of arrows that were slung at this paper) and it was evident that perhaps it was not statistically significant. So people started going off in all directions trying to find out what was important – oestrogen or orchiectomy, and in which sequence. Well, now the V. A. study has attempted to create some order out of this chaos, and I think that they are doing a very good job of it. I think that it is premature to say that patients are definitely going to live longer, or as long, with placebo, as they would on oestrogen therapy from the time the diagnosis is made. The trend though seems to be well-established. I think they have certainly pointed out the hazards of oestrogen therapy in patients who are poor risk cardiacs, or who have some element of cardiac disease. So I for one am watching the V. A. study very carefully.

C. V. Hodges: I think that I have made two important alterations in my treatment regimen as a result of the study. I no longer use 5 mg of stilboestrol but will stick to 1 mg, and I won't start therapy with oestrogen until symptoms appear. I think time alone will help us to determine whether the study was actually, in truth, what it was reported to be.

R. H. Flocks: I roughly agree with Dr. *Brendler,* having had this kind of experience which some of the rest of us have here. We wish to congratulate Dr. *Mellinger* and the Veterans group for doing a cooperative study so extensively. Now this is a very difficult thing to do, and I think Dr. *Mellinger* is to be congratulated upon being able to get such a group to work together. There are so many individuals who want to do things individually in the various parts of our country.

W. E. Goodwin: Dr. *Flocks,* has this altered your thinking or treatment in any way?

R. H. Flocks: It has reinforced the original opinion which Dr. *Alcock* had, that we should put off oestrogen therapy until the patient shows symptoms.

W. W. Scott: I have always reserved endocrine therapy for a late stage and on a small dose, so this has not changed anything really, as far as that is concerned. These studies are extremely difficult to conduct. I think that there are at least four of us in the room who were members of the old Cancer Chemotherapy National Survey Centre Study. That study was abandoned because the NIH told us that our statistician was too strict. Our statistician was *Donald Maitland,* one of the finest people in the business. This was the reason why the study was terminated. I don't know anything about statistics but some of the data is a little worrisome to me. I think that it should be made available to people, in detail, so that it would be possible for one to take as close a look as one wanted. This is what I would like to do.

W. Brosig: I am not very satisfied because we still don't know what we should do in case of cancer of the prostate. If we accept the work of *Mellinger* and his co-workers as a basis we are left in a dilemma. We have different stages. He does only differ 4 groups whilst we are regarding 5 groups here, but I think that does not matter. If there is an operable case, according to the groups I and perhaps II, we have to do total prostatectomy. The question is what to do in groups III and IV. Group IV are the cases who are in a bad condition. So we should treat them according to your findings with oestrogen, because oestrogen is at least as good as orchiectomy. I get the impression that we should not do orchiectomy any more. The question is only what to do in group III? Patients who have got cancer with nodes and maybe with bony metastases and who have no complaints; or you have a patient of group C without metastases. May you dare not treat him, because half a year later he could have metastases?

G. T. Mellinger: This has been a 6 year follow-up on most of our patients – some of them are a 10 year follow-up. I have just presented Dr. *Scott* with the crude figures. Following these patients up with an average follow-up of 6 years, we have about the same number of metastases in those who are on stilboestrol, as those who are on placebo.

Frequency of prostatic cancer

W. E. Goodwin: One of the questions that we have been asked is something about statistics of prostatic cancer in the United States. I am going to ask: How many new cases of prostatic cancer can be expected to turn up each year in the United States?

W. W. Scott: The most recent figures were compiled by the U.S. Health Service for 10 major cities, maybe 4 or 5 years ago. Prostatic cancer led the list in incidence per 100 000 of the adult male population. In prevalence, that means the number of cancers known, plus the incidence of new cases, it again led the list. Unfortunately, I can not remember this figure. In terms of mortality it was second to carcinoma of the lung and bronchus, but greater than any other carcinoma of any one portion of the bowel — stomach, colon or rectum — but, not all of those tumours combined. It was the second most common cancer.

R. H. Flocks: As I recall, the figure in 1968 was 14000 deaths from carcinoma of the prostate in the United States. It was the leading cause of death in males over the age of 65, as far as cancer is concerned.

W. E. Goodwin: In our Veterans'Hospital in Los Angeles, every eleventh patient that comes into the Urology ward has a cancer of the prostate. One patient in 11.

W. Brosig: I have here the death rate in Germany of 1967-68. There were 64000 men who died of cancer. 5000 of these died from prostatic cancer, that is the third place in the list, concerning death from cancer.

Early diagnosis of prostatic cancer

W. E. Goodwin: Another question is: "How do you go about finding cases which are in group A?" What is the best way to get cases like that? We know from the Hopkin's series that it is less than 10 % of prostatic cancers; more likely about 5 % fall into group A. These are surgically treatable. Dr. *Hodges,* how do you look for group A patients?

C. V. Hodges: It has been shown in the statistics from the armed services that one finds these early cases only by routine rectal examination of all males over 40. That is, their % was around 40 - 50 % of group A, or at least group A and B, whereas the figures are otherwise 5 - 10 %, as you stated. In Oregon for some reason Dr. *Mellinger* tells me, we have a higher % of goup B lesions in the Veteran's study — around 40 % — than any other group. I have been racking my brain to try to explain this. I cannot do it.

W. E. Goodwin: Dr. *Scott* would you like to tell us how to find a group A patient?

W. W. Scott: By routine rectal palpation. What really distresses me in this whole business is that I am sure that prostatic cancer has to begin as a small focus of cancer. It has to start somewhere and therefore it should start as a nodule. I presume that you ought to be able to feel about 1/2 of these, because prostatic cancer arises in the outer prostate in 99 % of the cases. 1/2 of these are in the posterior lamella, not the lateral lamella of the outer lobe. So you ought to be able to feel these, and yet the killing cancers that we see, just seem to spring from nowhere. This is my own personal experience with a number of members from the Faculty who had routine rectal examination and turned úp the next year with a disseminated cancer. This is really what distresses me about the whole business. I think we don't know enough about the natural history of the nodules themselves — these well-differentiated nodules. We do know, from the work of *Sam Franks* and others, that as we grow older — our chances of having a cancer get greater and greater. But also as we grow older and older, the chances that we'll have a well differentiated cancer grow better and better. I think that the killing cancer, at a mean age of 64, is a different cancer from the well-differentiated, isolated, palpable prostatic nodule.

Prevention of suspected cardio-vascular complications

W. E. Goodwin: One of the questions was: "How can one prevent vascular problems when a patient has to be treated this way? " For example, let's say, you have somebody who has a history of coronary disease, who is in partial cardiac failure with ankle oedema, and you find that you must treat him for a widespread prostatic cancer. Dr. *Mellinger* would you speak on that subject?

G. T. Mellinger: We have been using various treatments with these patients, and we have substantially reduced the cardiovascular mortality in study II, since we found out about this from study I. These patients receive good medical care by the internists. These patients are put on Diu or other diuretics. They usually receive one of the digitalis preparations, or they may receive quinidine or some such drug. It has been suggested that possibly all patients who receive oestrogens should at the same time receive diuretics. I think this might be a very good idea, particularly if they have a history of previous heart disease.

W. W. Scott: You mean all your patients are pretreated with digoxin or quinidine?

G. T. Mellinger: Only those with heart disease.

W. W. Scott: How do you double blind this in your evaluation, and comparison of heart disease with or without treatment?

G. T. Mellinger: All of the patients who have any sort of a heart disease receive the full medical treatment. Some of these will not receive stilboestrol, some do. Their needs for digoxin are probably greater when they are on higher doses of stilboestrol.

W. E. Goodwin: As we want to know what is the German attitude about the V. A. study, and about prostatic cancer, we would like to ask Prof. *Brosig* to summarise that for us.

W. Brosig: The German standpoint was that we had to try finding out what your standpoint is. That is the reason why we invited you. But I will give you a short summary of the present situation: The treatment of prostatic carcinoma in Germany is based on Huggins' work and his publications. This means that only a few clinics do a total prostatectomy in Germany today. Oestrogens and similar substances, with a dose of 2—5 mg daily, are given until the end of life. Since the publication of the Veterans Hospital study, everybody has been made uncertain. During the last 2 days we tried to find out, really, what treatment should be used. From *Mellinger's* figures the conclusion seemed clear to me. I would like to ask for the figures of the "big shots" we have invited here, as we don't know until now exactly what therapy should be done.

Groups I and II form only 10 % of all patients. According to *Mellinger's* figures, oestrogen is indicated only in group IV. We want to find out what all of you will do in group III.

There's also a question about orchiectomy. Should it be done or not? Who does it, and why does he still do it? Another question is — "If oestrogens are so harmful, why couldn't we give cyproterone acetate or progesterins instead?" This is a question we have to discuss. So when we close this conference we should know more than when we started.

E. Schmiedt: I have two questions for the panel. The 1st question is for Prof. *Kaufman.* Yesterday, Prof. *Kaufman* said that he, in stage III and IV performed an orchiectomy and oestrogen therapy. The day before we heard from Prof. *Scott* the orchiectomy effect will be over three months later. I want to ask, why do you still perform orchiectomy?

Testosterone shock therapy

The other question is, has anybody experience with the androgen shock therapy. In 4 extreme cases stage IV — we gave 100 mg. of testosterone daily for a week and afterwards we adminstered high doses of oestrogen — Honvan.

W. E. Goodwin: Dr. *Brendler,* are you ready to speak about the question of testosterone shock therapy which was raised by Prof. *Schmiedt?*

H. Brendler: Well I don't know if I can answer this question completely. I don't know if I have all the information necessary, but briefly, the effect of testosterone in prostatic cancer was reported by *Huggins* in one of his early papers. He simply stated that testosterone excited the prostatic cancer. It made it grow more rapidly. Following that there was no work done in this field until 1947 or 1948 when Dr. *Scott,* Dr. *Chase* and myself used testosterone in several patients with this disease, in Baltimore.

The first patient was a very interesting one. He developed a serious reactivation, following the use of testosterone, and this was so severe that he had to be hospitalised. After he recovered, following the use of large doses of stilboestrol, he was again started on testosterone. This is something that, I'm sure, would not be done today but at that time we were very interested in exploring the effects of testosterone, and to our amazement this patient had a very gratifying subjective response. I emphasise the word *subjective.* Certainly his bone pain lessened. His serum acid phosphatase rose to extremely high levels, but he felt better — there was no question about it. Now this was the same patient who about 1 month earlier had suffered *extremely* severe pain following the use of testosterone propionate, 100 mg daily, intramuscularly. We studied three more patients and we reported on these patients in the Journal of the American Medical Association in 1949. We observed two of these patients. Despite the fact that the serum acid phosphatase levels rose to very high levels, they improved subjectively. In neither of these patients was there any evidence of prostatic growth. In the 3rd patient who had a normal serum acid phosphatase level to begin with, the values of serum acid phosphatase did not change. Now following this initial study several other investigators used testosterone, and in general, the results were as follows. About 5 % of the patients developed reactivation — a serious excitation of their disease. In another 5 or 10 % there was a subjective improvement, and this, one would expect, as a result of the anabolic effects of testosterone. In the other 80 % there was no response. I think this experience has been the general one, from people who have written about it, and who have discussed it at meetings. Lastly, the cooperative study group utilised testosterone in a double blind clinical trial. The testosterone was administered in doses of 100 mg 3 times a week and the other unknown drug was stilboestrol which was given in doses of 10 mg 3 times a week. These 2 drugs were used in patients who had reactivated prostatic cancer. This means patients who had previously been treated and who had either had a response or not, but who were now in the last stages of the disease. I can report to you that in approx. 200 patients there was no response to either testosterone or stilboestrol. There were a few patients in whom the response was questionable but in the eyes of the statisticians who analysed our figures, there were no responses either good or bad following the use of testosterone.

TREATMENT — INDIVIDUAL PROCEEDING

Staging

W. E. Goodwin: One of the things that caused some confusion was that we had 5 groups of cancer instead of 4. Our German colleagues are accustomed to using 4. We point out that this staging which Dr. *Flocks* has given us is based on knowledge gained in the operating room. This means that there you can find out whether the patient has nodes or not. So we are going to abandon this 5 grouping which is a staging based on the operating room, and go back to the 4 stages.

Occult carcinoma

According to this staging (which is the one we use at UCLA)[1,2]), A and B are curable by surgery, and C and D are not curable. We're going to ask each member of the panel to tell us how he would treat each one of these types of cancer. But before we do that, there was still another type which wasn't mentioned and should have been mentioned yesterday. It is when an occult cancer, which is not palpable, nor suspected, is discovered by accident in a transurethral, or any kind of a prostate specimen, removed for benign hypertrophy. So the first question I'm going to ask you is, if we had an accidental discovery of a single focus of prostatic cancer in a transurethral specimen, how would you treat that patient?

J. J. Kaufman: I think a lot depends upon whether the occult carcinoma is in one focus, or multifocal. If it's in one focus of an adenoma, and in one area − I'd do nothing.

C. V. Hodges: I would agree.

H. Brendler: I would carry out prompt total prostatectomy.

R. H. Flocks: I would find out whether there is more carcinoma in the capsule, by biopsy transurethrally of the capsule. If there is carcinoma, I would treat it aggressively either by radiation or by radical prostatectomy.

W. W. Scott: A total prostatectomy via the perineum.

W. Brosig: We don't treat them at all.

W. E. Goodwin: We are now posed the same question. You've found a transurethral specimen which has multiple foci. Unexpectedly you find that there are many foci of prostatic cancer. Dr. *Kaufman?*

J. J. Kaufman: And that's unsuspected clinically. I would do a total prostatectomy − prostatovesiculectomy, either by the perineal or retropubic route.

C. V. Hodges: I would also do a total prostatectomy.

H. Brendler: The same.

R. H. Flocks: The same.

W. W. Scott: The same.

W. Brosig: Up to now we did orchiectomy and oestrogen therapy.

Stage A cancer

W. E. Goodwin: Now I'm going to ask the panel to look at group A, which is a clinical staging based on finding a nodule at rectal examination. You don't know what it is but you feel something hard in that area. What do you do in this circumstance, Dr. *Kaufman?*

---

[1]) *Goodwin, W. E.:* Discussion of Paper by: *Presti, J. C.:* Carcinoma of the prostate; Diagnosis and Treatment, California Medicine 78, 443, May 1953.

[2]) *Kaufman, J. J., Rosenthal, M.* and *Goodwin, W. E.:* Methods of Diagnosis of Carcinoma of the Prostate: A Comparison of Clinical Impression, Prostatic Smear, Needle Biopsy, Open Perineal Biopsy and Transurethal Biopsy. Journal of Urology 72, 450−465, September 1954.

J. J. Kaufman: I'd do a total prostatectomy, either perineal or retropubic.

W. E. Goodwin: Wouldn't you want to find out if it's a cancer first?

J. J. Kaufman: Oh! I'm assuming that we've proven it's a cancer.

W. E. Goodwin: How would you prove it?

J. J. Kaufman: I, personally, use a needle biopsy in these cases, unless I am extremely suspicious of the lesion. If the man is a candidate for a perineal operation, on the basis of his body build and my own desire to do a perineal rather than a retropubic prostatectomy, I would do an open perineal biopsy and proceed directly. If I had made the decision in advance that I wanted to do a retropubic operation on this man, I would do a needle biopsy through the perineum. If that came back negative, I would then proceed to do an open perineal biopsy, should my index of suspicion be high enough.

C. V. Hodges: I would do an open perineal biopsy, and a radical prostatectomy, preferably perineally, but if it looked as though it would be difficult, I would convert to a radical retropubic.

H. Brendler: I would do an open perineal biopsy, and a total perineal prostatectomy, if the frozen section were positive. I would offer a strong *no* to needle biopsy. I think the results are very misleading, and I want the patient in the operating room when I biopsy that prostate.

W. E. Goodwin: You know, yesterday, you said that it was obvious that I was a Brendler-trained man. I find myself in total agreement with what you've just said.

R. H. Flocks: There are several factors to consider. First the age. If the patient is over 75 years of age, in our modern society, I would probably make a diagnosis, preferably by a needle biopsy, or I might even observe the patient, and continue to do nothing other than simply observe him. If he's under 75, I would expose the prostate perineally, get a definitive diagnosis, and if the lesion was exactly as it's shown in that slide, I would do a total perineal prostatectomy. Now if, in addition to his being under 75, he's in his early 60's and he has a good life expectancy, I would expose his lower abdomen three months later and do a lymphadenectomy.

W. W. Scott: I have little to add except to emphasise the importance of doing a biopsy, and in our country, often enough, the patient does not have a biopsy before he is treated hormonally. He always has a biopsy before he's treated by an open prostatectomy. In a series of 209 nodules in our hospital, biopsied via the perineum — 108 were cancers, 111 were *not* cancers, and in a retrospective study of the charts, it was not possible to determine which ones were cancers, and which were not cancers. They were equally distributed between the apical, median and basal portions of the gland. Their consistency was similar in many instances. I would really like to emphasise the importance of this.

W. Brosig: Usually, if the patient was less than 70 years of age we did an open perineal biopsy, and a perineal prostatectomy. Now I will extend the age to 75, I think, from what I have heard and seen here. Only if the findings were not clear, or we didn't intend to do a radical operation we would do a needle biopsy.

W. E. Goodwin: We see then that there's a difference of opinion amongst the panel as to whether needle biopsy or open biopsy should be done. I suppose it is a personal preference. I feel that a needle biopsy is not reliable enough (if it comes back negative) to say — all right the patient does not have a cancer. So I feel that in either A or B, you must do an open biopsy to answer that question.

J. J. Kaufman: May I have one remark. Dr. *Goodwin's* name is on a paper that states that needle biopsy is a very satisfactory procedure. However, I feel that like anything else a needle biopsy in the hands of someone who is very experienced in doing needle biopsies is much more reliable than in the hands of someone who doesn't have a lot of experience with a biopsy of this type. I feel that if you get tissue back which explains why this patient has an area of induration, and by that, I mean you get — "fibromuscular stroma, suggesting a leiomyoma", or "granuloma suggesting either tuberculous or other types of granulomatous prostatitis" — then you can be reasonably satisfied that you have explained this patient's area of induration. If you get back — "adenomatous tissue", or "normal tissues" — then it behooves you to get either another needle biopsy or do an open perineal biopsy. Most of the time we can be reasonably sure of the diagnosis even though Dr. *Scott* would take issue with this. I feel that a man who comes in with a nodule gives me an impression of having a carcinoma or not. Some are very, very suspicious and you know it's going to be carcinoma, and you're not satisfied until you've absolutely proven that it's not. Others are just little areas of induration at the base of the prostate, and you hesitate to expose this man's prostate to an open perineal biopsy, when this in a young man carries at least a 30 % risk of impotence.

Timing of radical prostatectomy

W. E. Goodwin: We still have to go back once more to a finding of occult carcinoma unexpected in a transurethral specimen. There's another question which has come up, which is this: 'Assuming that you find multiple foci, and assuming that you're going to do radical prostatectomy, when do you do it? ' When in time, in relation to the transurethral biopsy?

R. H. Flocks: I like to wait until the prostatic urethra is healed, following prostatectomy. My pathological studies have shown that this takes anywhere from 6—8 weeks. So I wait 2 months.

W. W. Scott: No addition.

W. Brosig: If we did a transurethral before, we always treat the patient conservatively, not by a radical prostatectomy any more.

H. Brendler: I go ahead immediately.

C. V. Hodges: I would go ahead as soon as I could get the patient on the surgical schedule.

J. J. Kaufman: I would go ahead immediately.

W. E. Goodwin: I can't resist referring to a paper that I wrote about 20 years ago, called 'Radical Prostatectomy After Previous Prostatic Surgery.' It's in the JAMA, and it seemed from a study of cases which I made at Johns Hopkins, that after transurethral, it didn't make any difference when you did the radical prostatectomy. You could go ahead soon or late. But if it was being done after a supra-pubic or retropubic prostatectomy, you had better wait at least 6—8 weeks, or else the operation would be unsuccessful.

Stage B cancer

Now we'll go on with Group B which is a little more advanced, but still limited to the prostate (at least I take it to be that) and therefore still curable I would ask each member of the panel how he would treat this condition?

J. J. Kaufman: We assume now that the biopsy is established. I would do a total prostatectomy by either route.

C. V. Hodges: I would do the same.

H. Brendler: The same.

R. H. Flocks: I would expose the prostate perineally and plan to do a total prostatectomy. I would be ready to infiltrate the bed of the prostate with a radioactive material, or seriously consider postoperative radiation therapy, because as we showed on the 1st day in the pathological studies of Dr. *Mostofi* and as I showed yesterday, the incidence of local recurrence due to microscopic extension here is high. Moreover in younger patients, in their sixties with a long life expectancy, if there is any microscopic extension, or even without microscopic extension, the incidence of lymph node involvement is substantial. Therefore, I would do a lower abdominal exploration, and a lymphadenectomy, 2 months later.

W. W. Scott: I would probably attempt a total perineal prostatectomy, but I'd be a little worried by that lesion which *looks* as extensive as it is.

W. Brosig: I will do a radical prostatectomy.

Stage C cancer

W. E. Goodwin: Now we come to Group C, which has extended beyond the prostate on the seminal vesicles, and possibly laterally towards the levator muscles. In other words it has extended beyond the prostate itself. Dr. *Kaufman?*

J. J. Kaufman: Now we're getting into the Group that Dr. *Schmiedt* referred to, and I think that perhaps he misunderstood me when I said that I do orchiectomy on these groups C and D. What I implied was that things were reasonably clear to us, 10 or 15 years ago, at which time these lesions were treated by orchiectomy and 5 mg of stilboestrol, but now because of the tremendous number of choices that we have, we find ourselves very much in limbo, as to whether to employ orchiectomy or oestrogen, or both, or cyproterone, or radiation therapy or what. Now getting to Group C it would depend on whether this man had obstructive urinary symptoms. If he had obstructive urinary symptoms I would treat him with a transurethral resection. I would guess that he has no elevation of his acid phosphatase, and he has no positive nodes or bone lesions. So that's all I would do for this man, and then I would watch him very carefully. If the lesion began to grow, it could obstruct again quickly, then I would treat this man with local irradiation, like cobalt.

W. E. Goodwin: One of the questions which was asked and spoken about, but the answer was not understood, is — If you had such a patient in Group C, and you treated him with oestrogens, and then in 6 months you examined him, and you couldn't feel the cancer anymore, would you then do a total prostatectomy?

J. J. Kaufman: Well I have done this. I don't think I can say that I can be doctrinaire in this respect. I would say that if this type of patient is young, if he has a good life expectancy, I might do a radical prostatectomy on this type of patient, after he has made a good response to oestrogen therapy. What I'm saying is that this is a contradiction to what I've just said, because I said earlier that I would not treat this man with oestrogens, *preferentially.* I would do a TUR if he was obstructed, and give him radiation therapy. We can go on to say that if this man responded to radiation therapy, I would not give him 7000 rads, if I were considering a prostatectomy subsequently, then I would consider doing a total prostatectomy on this man. I would have had to make up my mind in advance as to whether I wanted to do a prostatectomy on this man or not. There are many shades that you have to consider in the decision.

H. Brendler: I would carry out castration immediately, place the patient on stilboestrol, 5 mg daily, and I would irradiate the prostate. We've been doing that for the past year.

R. H. Flocks: Group C presents a real problem as Dr. *Kaufman* emphasised. I think we need to emphasise that ablation therapy, and by ablation therapy I mean surgery or irradiation, is not contradictory to the simultaneous utilisation, or the utilisation in the future of other types of endocrine manipulation. These 2 treatments are not mutually exclusive. It has been emphasised by some of the speakers today, that there is certainly a group of cells in this tumour that are not androgen dependent. So the attempts to destroy these are certainly in order, in the correct case. Now, if a man is over 70 or over 75, whichever age you want to empirically utilise as the dividing point, I believe that treatment for obstruction and endocrine manipulation is in order. As you noted there is a difference of opinion with regard to the timing of the endocrine manipulation. Our own feeling is that if there are no symptoms whatsoever, we don't start the endocrine manipulation until later. On the other hand if this patient is younger, and virile, my policy is to do radical surgery plus irradiation. As I showed you yesterday in 90-odd cases that have been followed for 10 years, there were only 4 local recurrences. Now the interesting thing about those 90 cases is, that over 80 % of them at the end of 5 years showed no evidence of metastasis. The quality of their survival was excellent. However by the 8th year, many of these began to show evidence of bone metastasis. Not in every one of the 91, but in many of these, I did do pelvic lymphadenectomy, and in the 75 % of the patients who had positive nodes, they lived past 5 years and were well, but then in the period between the 5th and 10th year they began to show evidence of metastasis, at which time we began to treat them with the various forms of endocrine manipulation.

W. W. Scott: I would like to emphasise, again, my feeling about the importance of adding histological grading to staging, because I think this is an extremely important consideration. I think that this is the only way in which we are going to be able to evaluate these different modalities of treatment. I would also like to emphasise, in reporting, that one compares pure treatments with pure treatments. By that I mean, compare orchiectomy with orchiectomy and not with a combination of orchiectomy and radiation therapy, and analyse your results in terms of orchiectomy, or radiation therapy. If we mix up the treatment, we are never going to learn the effect of the particular form of treatment that we are using. There has been great confusion in this regard. You asked earlier about whether or not one could make an inoperable prostatic cancer operable. Well there are figures in the American literature which indicate that you can. But in that paper there is no indication as to the grade of the tumour that we are dealing with, and I think that it would make a great deal of difference, whether there were well differentiated or poorly differentiated tumours.

Again I'd emphasise that in our own series of nodules, and I'm talking only about nodules, that if the grade of the tumour was high, none of these people were free of cancer 15 years later. If the tumour had extended to perivescular fascia, because prostatic cancer doesn't extend to the seminal vesicles per se, then there were no cures.

W. Brosig: Until now we did orchiectomy and we gave oestrogens. If the tumour was widespread, we also gave radiation therapy sometimes. If there were obstructive symptoms, we waited. We didn't do a transurethral straight away, because we think it is dangerous to do a TUR in an untreated cancer. I have no experience, but I would like to know your answer to this point. What I shall do now, I don't know.

W. E. Goodwin: The person who asked the question about doing prostatectomy after giving oestrogens, wanted to know the results, and rather than take the few remaining minutes, I will give 3 references that I know of. There are probably others. The first one is by *Colston* and *Brendler* from Johns Hopkins. The second by *Chute* of Boston. And the third by *Winfield W. Scott.* The other *W. W. Scott,* the *Rochester Scott.*

Stage D cancer

In each case there seemed to be some results that were good, but as Dr. *Scott* (the *Baltimore Scott*) says, it didn't tell us about the type of the tumour. Now we have just a few remaining moments, so we'll finally come to Group D, and ask each member of the panel, "If you have a locally extensive cancer, with evidence of bony metastases and you don't know, whether there are nodes or not but you can fairly assume that there are, how do you treat Group D? "

C. V. Hodges: I would assume that this is a symptomatic patient. My preference would be to start him on stilboestrol. For the time being, I think, we don't know enough about cyproterone acetate, we just don't know enough about it to include it in our discussion right now.

W. E. Goodwin: If you had a choice between stilboestrol and cyproterone, which would you use?

C. V. Hodges: I haven't been able to make up my mind, as yet, on the basis of our experience.

W. E. Goodwin: What dose of stilboestrol would you use?

C. V. Hodges: I think here, Dr. *Staehler* has a point, in that one can start with a higher dose. We'll say 5 mg t.i.d. (tres in die) which is not massive at all, but this could be continued from 2–4 weeks, and then I would drop it to 1 mg daily. I would continue the patient on this, until he had a relapse and then I would do an orchiectomy.

W. E. Goodwin: We haven't got enough time to spend on dosage but Dr. *Belt* told me, after what he said about the 300 mg a day, that he had discussed this subject with Dr. *Fergusson* from London who agreed completely with Dr. *Belt's* experience. Dr. *Brendler* how would you treat Group D?

H. Brendler: I would carry out prompt castration. Up until this morning I would have placed the patient on stilboestrol 5 mg daily, but I was also very impressed with Dr. *Staehler's* point, and I am going to give this more thought. I think there is something to this. In addition to castration and stilboestrol, I would irradiate painful metastases which did not respond to the *Endocrine* therapy.

J. J. Kaufman: I am in perfect agreement with Dr. *Hodges.*

R. H. Flocks: I'm in agreement with Dr. *Hodges.*

W. W. Scott: Nothing to add.

W. Brosig: We always did orchiectomy, and we gave 1000 mg Honvan daily during the 1st week and then we switched over to Depot estradiol, 100 mg every 3 weeks. But I still want to ask whether we should still do orchiectomy or not?

W. W. Scott: I certainly believe in this form of treatment. Without question.

R. H. Flocks: Yes. I have found, as I'm sure most of you have, that peculiarly enough, changing the type of drug, or adding, as Dr. *Hodges* mentioned, orchiectomy, often produces a new remission.

I was very much interested in Dr. *Schmiedt's* remarks on Honvan. I have used this to a great extent, and in a very substantial number of patients this has produced a new remission. We, about 15 years ago, gave 17 consecutive patients testosterone. Four of these patients developed a markedly elevated acid — phosphatase and marked symptoms. These responded more rapidly to Honvan than those others, who had not got this markedly deleterious effect from testosterone.

W. E. Goodwin: The question is, do you believe in orchiectomy?

H. Brendler: Ardently. I firmly believe in orchiectomy.

C. V. Hodges: Yes, I believe in orchiectomy.

W. E. Goodwin: Castration without representation.

J. J. Kaufman: Yes, I believe in orchiectomy too, but I use it as an "ace in the hole" these days. I think it does give a very good remission. I think it is better than doing the reverse. In other words, using orchiectomy at the outset and keeping stilboestrol for later or other types of female hormones, or using both of them together. I think it is nice, to have orchiectomy as an "ace in the hole", because usually after patients have escaped from control with female hormones (with progestational agents), then what we can do is to give them at least a year in some cases, with an orchiectomy. —

W. E. Goodwin: Well, I think we have done our duty. I wish to express my appreciation to the panel and to the audience. And I think we all express our appreciation to Schering A. G. and Asta Werke A. G. I would like now to thank you for allowing me to participate.

Closing Addresses

W. Brosig and H. Brendler *)

Urologische und Poliklinik im Klinikum Steglitz der Freien Universität Berlin, Germany

*) Department of Urology, The Mt. Sinai Hospital, New York, N. Y., USA

W. Brosig: The time has come to close the session. I would like to say "many thanks" to *Willard Goodwin* who made such a good moderator, and helped us to perform this meeting. I also would like to thank Prof. *Kramer,* Dr. *Bernhard,* Dr. *Friedrichs* from the Schering AG, and all of the others who helped us so much. Special thanks to Dr. *Baumgärtel* who made all the arrangements. Last, not least, I like to thank all the fine colleagues from abroad, and from Germany, who were so ardent participants of this symposium. I can only say: "Auf Wiedersehen in Berlin!"

H. Brendler: I thank this meeting. As one of the participants, I should like to join with the others in thanking the Schering AG for making all this possible.

I thank Dr. *Brosig* for organising this meeting in such expert fashion, and esp. to Dr. *Goodwin,* who, I think, deserves a vote of thanks from all of us, for handling this meeting in such a fine manner. He has made possible the exchange of opinions which has come about during the past 3 days, and made it possible for some fruitful discussion.

Participants

Alken, C. E., Prof. Dr. med.,
Direktor der Urologischen Univ.-Klinik
665 Homburg (Saar)

Bagshaw, M. A., M. D. Prof. and Director
Division of Radiation Therapy
Stanford University School of Medicine
Stanford, Calif., 94305

Balogh, F., Prof. Dr.,
Pecs, Munkascy M. u. Z.

Baumgärtel, H., Dr. med.,
Oberarzt der Urologischen Klinik und
Poliklinik im Klinikum Steglitz
der Freien Universität Berlin
1 Berlin 45, Hindenburgdamm 30

Belt, E., M. D., B. A., M. S., M. D., L. O. D.
Clinical Prof. of Surgery (Urology)
UCLA School of Med.
1893 Wilshire Boulevard, Los Angeles, Calif.
90057

Bischoff, P., Prof. Dr.,
Chefarzt der Urologischen Abteilung
Elisabeth-Krankenhaus
2 Hamburg 20

Brendler, H., Dr.,
Department of Urology
Prof. and Chairman The Mt. Sinai Hospital
100th Street and Fifth Avenue New York,
N. Y. 10029

Briggs, M. H., Prof. Dr.,
Director of Research and Development
Schering Chemicals Ltd.
Victoria Way, Burgess Hill, Sussex

Brock, N., Prof. Dr. med.,
Leiter der Pharmakol. Abteilung
ASTA-Werke AG
4812 Brackwede

Brosig, W., Prof. Dr. med.,
Direktor der Urologischen Klinik und Poliklinik im Klinikum Steglitz der Freien Universität Berlin
1 Berlin 45, Hindenburgdamm 30

Büscher, H. K., Prof. Dr.
Leit. Arzt d. Urologischen Abt. des Friederi-
kenstiftes
3 Hannover

Burkert, H., Dr. med.,
ASTA-Werke AG
4814 Senne I, Berliner Str. 69

Coolsaet, B., Dr.
Urolog. Department
De Wever Ziekenhuis
Henri-Dunant-Str., Heerlen, Holland

Dettmar, H., Prof. Dr. med.,
Direktor der Urologischen Univ.-Klinik
4 Düsseldorf, Moorenstraße 5

Dierking, K., Dr. med.,
ASTA-Werke AG
4812 Brackwede

Fergusson, J. D.,
82 Portland Place, London W. I.

Flocks, R. H., M. D.
Prof. of Urology University Hospital
Iowa City, Iowa 52240

Frick, J., Dr. med.,
Urologische Univ.-Klinik
Innsbruck

Friedrichs, M., M. D.
Berlin Laboratories
445 Park Avenue, New York, N. Y. 10022

Frohmüller, H., Priv. Doz. Dr. med.,
Leiter d. Urol. Abt. d. Chirurg. Univ.-Klinik
87 Würzburg, Staatl. Luitpoldkrankenhaus

Gaca, A. H., Dozent Dr. med.,
Leiter der Urolog. Abtlg.
Chirurg. Univ.-Klinik
78 Freiburg i. Br., Hugstetter Straße 55

Goodwin, W. E., Prof., M. D.
Director of Division of Urology
The Center of the Health Sciences, University
of California
Los Angeles / Calif. 90024

Grayhack, J. T., M.D.
Prof. and Chairman Northwestern University
Medical School
303 E. Chicago Avenue, Chicago, Illinois 60611

Hauge, A., Dr. med.,
Oberarzt der Urologischen Klinik und Poliklinik im Klinikum Westend
der Freien Universität Berlin
1 Berlin 19, Spandauer Damm 130

Hodges, C. V., M. D.
UOMS
3181 S. W. Sam Jackson Park Road, Portland,
Oregon 97201

Hohenfellner, R., Prof. Dr.,
Direktor der Urologischen Klinik der
Joh. Gutenberg-Universität
65 Mainz, Langenbeckstraße 1

Jönsson, G., Prof. Dr.,
Urologiska Universitetskliniken
Lund

Kaufman, J., M. D.
Prof. of Surgery / Urology, Ucla School of
Medicine
Los Angeles, Calif. 90024

Kelâmi, A., Dr.
Urol. Klinik und Poliklinik im
Klinikum Steglitz der Freien Universität Berlin
1 Berlin 45, Hindenburgdamm 30

Klosterhalfen, Prof. Dr.,
Direktor der Urolog. Univ.-Klinik,
Univ.-Krankenhaus Eppendorf
2 Hamburg 20, Martinistraße 52

Kollwitz, A. A., Prof. Dr.,
Urol. Klinik und Poliklinik im Klinikum
Steglitz der Freien Universität Berlin
1 Berlin 45, Hindenburgdamm 30

Kramer, M., Prof. Dr. med.,
Leiter der exp. med. Forschung der
Schering AG
1 Berlin 65, Müllerstr. 170−172

Lutzeyer, W., Prof. Dr. med.,
Ordentlicher Professor für Urologie der
Medizinischen Fakultät der Rhein.-West.
Techn. Hochschule
51 Aachen, Goethestraße 27/29

McDonald, D. F., M.D.
Prof. and Chief, Division of Urology
Galveston, Texas 77550

Marberger, H., Prof. Dr. med.,
Urologische Abteilung Chirurg. Univ.-Klinik
6020 Innsbruck

Mauermayer, W., Priv. Doz. Dr.,
Chefarzt d. Urolog. Klinik des Klinikums
rechts der Isar der TH München
8 München 80, Ismaningerstr. 22

Mellin, P., Prof. Dr. med.,
Direktor der Urologischen Klinik
Klinikum Essen der Ruhr-Universität Bochum
43 Essen, Hufelandstraße 55

Mellinger, G. T., M.D.
Chairman, Veterans Administration
Cooperative Urological Research Group,
Chief, Urology Section
Minneapolis, Minnesota 55417

Mostofi, F.K., Dr.
Armed Forces Institute of
Pathology
Washington, D.C. 20305

Nagamatsu, G. R., M.D.
Prof. of Urology
Department of Urology, New York
Medical College, Flower and Fifth Avenue
Hospitals
Fifth Avenue and 106th Street, New York,
N. Y. 10029

Nagel, R., Prof. Dr.,
Direktor der Urol. Klinik und Poliklinik
im Klinikum Westend der Freien Univ. Berlin
1 Berlin 19, Spandauer Damm 130

Neumann, F., Dr. med. vet.,
Leiter der Abt. für exp. Endokrinologie der
Schering AG
1 Berlin 65, Müllerstr. 170-172

Rodeck, Prof. Dr. med.
Abteilung f. Urologie der Universitäts-Klinik
355 Marburg (Lahn), Robert-Koch-Str. 8

Röhl, L., Prof. Dr.,
Leiter der Urol. Abt. Chirurgische Univ.-
Klinik
69 Heidelberg, Voss-Straße 2

Rothauge, C. F., Prof. Dr. med.,
Lehrstuhl und Abt. für Urologie
der Justus Liebig-Universität
63 Gießen

Salloch, R. R., Dr. med.,
Abt. f. experimentelle Endokrinologie der
Schering AG
1 Berlin 65, Müllerstraße 170-172

Schmiedt, E., Prof. Dr. med.
Direktor der Urol. Klinik und Poliklinik
der Universität München
8 München 15, Thalkirchner Straße 48

Schroeder, F., Dr. med., M.D.,
11088 Ophir Drive, Los Angeles, California
90024

Scott, Wm. W., Dr.,
Prof. of Urology, Hopkins Hospital
Baltimore/Maryland

Sigel, A., Prof. Dr.,
Urologische Abt. der Chirurgischen Univ.-
Klinik
852 Erlangen

Smith, R.B., M. D.,
Asst. Prof. Surgery/Urology, U. C. L. A.
Medical Center
Los Angeles, California 90024

Staehler, W., Prof. Dr.,
Chirurg. Klinik und Poliklinik der Universität Tübingen
74 Tübingen, Calwerstraße 7

Stoll, H. G., Dr. med.,
Direktor der Urol. Klinik Städt. Kranken-
anstalten Bremen
28 Bremen, St. Jürgen Straße

Straffon, R. A., M. D.,
Department of Urology, Cleveland Clinic
Cleveland/Ohio 44 106

Truss, F., Prof. Dr. med.,
Leiter der Urol. Abt. der Chirurg. Universitäts-Klinik
34 Göttingen, Goßlerstraße 10

Turner-Warwick, R. T., M. D.,
F.R.C.S., M.R., C.P.
61 Harley House, Marylebone Road,
London N.W. 1

Übelhör, R., Prof. Dr.,
Urologische Univ.-Klinik
1095 Wien, Alser Straße 4

Ufer, J., Dr. med.,
Abteilung Klinische Forschung der
Schering AG
1 Berlin 65, Müllerstr. 170-172

Veenema, R. J., M. D.,
Prof. of Clinical Urology, Chief of Urology
Francis Delafield Hospital Division,
Columbia University
New York, N. Y. 10032

Walsh, P., M. D.,
Dept. Surgery, Div. Urology UCLA School
of Medicine
Los Angeles, California 9024

Weber, W., Prof. Dr.,
Chirurgische Universitätsklinik
6 Frankfurt, Ludwig-Rahn-Str. 14

Williams, D. C., Dr., FRIC.,
The Marie Curie Memorial Foundation,
The Research Department, The Chart
Oxted, Surrey

Zingg, E., Prof. Dr. ,
Urologische Universitäts-Klinik
Rämistraße 100, 8000 Zürich

Name Index

» Advances in the Biosciences

Advances in the Biosciences 1
Schering Symposium on
Endocrinology, May 1967
1969 322 pp 235 ill.
ISBN 3 528 07680 1

Advances in the Biosciences 2
Schering Symposium on
Biodynamics and Mechanism of Action
of Steroid Hormones, March 1968
1969 353 pp. 213 ill.
ISBN 3 528 07681 X

Advances in the Biosciences 3
Schering Workshop on
Steroid Metabolism "In vitro
versus in vivo", December 1968
1969 217 pp 139 ill.
ISBN 3 528 07685 2

Advances in the Biosciences 4
Schering Symposium on
Mechanisms involved in Conception,
March 1969
1970 417 pp 289 ill.
ISBN 3 528 07686 0

Advances in the Biosciences 5
Schering Workshop on
Pharmacokinetics, May 1969
1970 285 pp 183 ill.
ISBN 3 528 07687 9

Advances in the Biosciences 6
Schering Symposium on
Intrinsic and Extrinsic Factors
Mammalian Development, April 1970
1971 656 pp 347 ill.
ISBN 3 528 07688 7

Advances in the Biosciences 7
Schering Workshop on
Steroid Hormone "Receptors",
December 1970
1971 approx. 460 pp
ISBN 3 528 07689 5

» Life Sciences Monographs

Life Sciences Monographs 1
International Symposium on
The Treatment of
Carcinoma of the Prostate
November 1969
1971 224 pp 145 ill.
ISBN 3 528 07811 1

Life Sciences Monographs 2
Schering Symposium über
Sexualdeviationen und
ihre medikamentöse Behandlung
Mai 1971
176 pp approx. 44 ill.
ISBN 3 528 07800 6

» **Life Sciences Monographs 2**

**Schering Symposium über
Sexualdeviationen und
ihre medikamentöse Behandlung
May 1971**

Editor: G. Laudahn. With ap. 44 ill. — New York / Braunschweig: Vieweg
1971. ap. VIII, 176 pages 15,5 x 21 cm.

ISBN 3 528 0**7800** 6

» **vieweg**